Nikolaos Konstantopoulos

Introduction to Biology

AF138541

Nikolaos Konstantopoulos

Introduction to Biology

LAP LAMBERT Academic Publishing

Impressum / Imprint
Bibliografische Information der Deutschen Nationalbibliothek: Die Deutsche Nationalbibliothek verzeichnet diese Publikation in der Deutschen Nationalbibliografie; detaillierte bibliografische Daten sind im Internet über http://dnb.d-nb.de abrufbar.
Alle in diesem Buch genannten Marken und Produktnamen unterliegen warenzeichen-, marken- oder patentrechtlichem Schutz bzw. sind Warenzeichen oder eingetragene Warenzeichen der jeweiligen Inhaber. Die Wiedergabe von Marken, Produktnamen, Gebrauchsnamen, Handelsnamen, Warenbezeichnungen u.s.w. in diesem Werk berechtigt auch ohne besondere Kennzeichnung nicht zu der Annahme, dass solche Namen im Sinne der Warenzeichen- und Markenschutzgesetzgebung als frei zu betrachten wären und daher von jedermann benutzt werden dürften.

Bibliographic information published by the Deutsche Nationalbibliothek: The Deutsche Nationalbibliothek lists this publication in the Deutsche Nationalbibliografie; detailed bibliographic data are available in the Internet at http://dnb.d-nb.de.
Any brand names and product names mentioned in this book are subject to trademark, brand or patent protection and are trademarks or registered trademarks of their respective holders. The use of brand names, product names, common names, trade names, product descriptions etc. even without a particular marking in this work is in no way to be construed to mean that such names may be regarded as unrestricted in respect of trademark and brand protection legislation and could thus be used by anyone.

Coverbild / Cover image: www.ingimage.com

Verlag / Publisher:
LAP LAMBERT Academic Publishing
ist ein Imprint der / is a trademark of
OmniScriptum GmbH & Co. KG
Bahnhofstraße 28, 66111 Saarbrücken, Deutschland / Germany
Email: info@lap-publishing.com

Herstellung: siehe letzte Seite /
Printed at: see last page
ISBN: 978-3-659-82385-5

Dedicated to my parents Konstantinos and Athina whose personal sacrifices allowed me to pursue my dreams. Dedicated also to my brother Ioannis for his support. Moreover dedicated to my professors for giving me the light of knowledge.

Table of contents

1) The cell

The cell was discovered by Robert Hooke and it is the basic functional, structural and reproductive unit of all the unicellular and multicellular organisms. It is a world on its own which is able to saw all the basic life manifestations (metabolism, growth, irritability, reproduction and development). The cells according to their structural characteristics and origin we can divide them into eukaryotic (animal and plant cells) and prokaryotic (bacteria). The prokaryotes where the first cell type that had appeared and their organization and structure is simpler than their eukaryotes counterparts.

PROKARYOTIC CELL

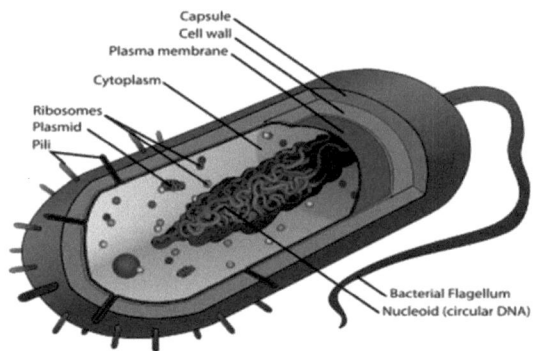

Structure and functions	Eukaryotic cells	Prokaryotic cells
Cell wall	Only in plant cells	Yes
Chloroplasts	Only in plant cells	No
Endoplasmic reticulum	Yes	No
Golgi apparatus	Yes	No
Intermediate filaments	Only in animal cells	No
Microfilaments	Yes	No
Microtubules	Yes	No
Mitochondria	Yes	No
Nuclear envelope	Yes	No
Nucleolus	Yes	No
Plasma membrane	Yes	Yes
Ribosomes	Yes	Yes
Size	10-100 μm diameter	0.1-5 μm diameter
Genetic-material	DNA combined with proteins	Naked DNA
Mitosis-Meiosis	Yes	No

The cell wall is located outside from the cell membrane and provides the cells with structural support and protection. We can found it in plants, bacteria, fungi. The major components of plant cell wall are long branched chains of the polysaccharide cellulose. In the cell wall of fungi we mainly find chitin which is a long-chain polymer of N-acetylglucosamine, a derivative of glucose. Some types of plant cells have an additional layer of protection from dehydration (due to hydrophobic character) and insults from insects. It is composed mainly from lipids and organic substances and it is the cerata, or waxes.

To the inside of a cell we can find a large proportion of water (40% of total body water of human body) which supports the survivor of cells and gives them their shape. This, in a way, leads to the compartmentalization of different subcellular components inside the membranous organelles of the cell, and protects them due to the hydrophobic character of their membranes.

The cytoskeleton of the cell is found from the inside part of the plasmatic membrane and its role is to maintain the cell's shape, anchors organelles in place, helps during endocytosis and exocytosis, and cytokinesis (separation of daughter cells after cell division). The eukaryotic cytoskeleton is composed mainly of microfilaments, intermediate filaments, microtubules and proteins.

Every cell type needs energy for survival and reproduction. In the human body every cell obtains the energy that needs through the oxidation of our foodstuffs (carbohydrates, proteins and lipids). Through the digestion, catabolism and oxidation of our foodstuffs are generated simple substances which enter the Krebs cycle, a metabolic pathway that generates the energy rich molecule of ATP (30,5 Kj/mol). ATP (adenosine triphosphate) is a universal donor of energy for living systems but not the only one. Inside the cells there are compounds with energy rich bonds in their molecules with a range of 30-60 Kj/mol.

1.1) Cell membrane

The plasmatic membrane is to separate the cell from its environment forming thus, two different worlds, the intracellular space and extracellular space. It is composed of a double layer of lipids which due to their hydrophobic character are aligned to the inside of the double layer, and hydrophilic phosphorus molecules facing the watery environment of the membrane. We speak thus for a phospholipid bilayer. Embedded in this membrane are also cholesterol and a variety of protein molecules that act as channels (porins) and pumps, which move different molecules into and out of the cell. That fluid mosaic model of membrane is semi-permeable because it permits to some molecules to enter or leave the cell, and others not. That is the basis of differentiation between intracellular fluid and extracellular fluid (the cell is in a higher energy state than its environment). The cell is not totally isolated from its environment and interacts with it. It will always try to be in equilibrium with its environment, but will never be. A cell that is in an absolute equilibrium with its environment is a non-living, dead cell.

Thus if we put an animal cell in a hypertonic solution, it will try to achieve an equal state with its environment. For this purpose it will lose water so as to dilute its environment, and as a consequence it will shrink and probably die. If we put a plant cell in a hypotonic solution, we must think of its cell wall. So, the cell again will try to be in equilibrium with its environment and will start the entry of water to the inside. This will not lead to any change of shape because it has the rigid cell wall. In the contrary, if we put the same cell in a hypertonic solution, it will start to lose water and the plasmatic membrane will detach from the cell wall.

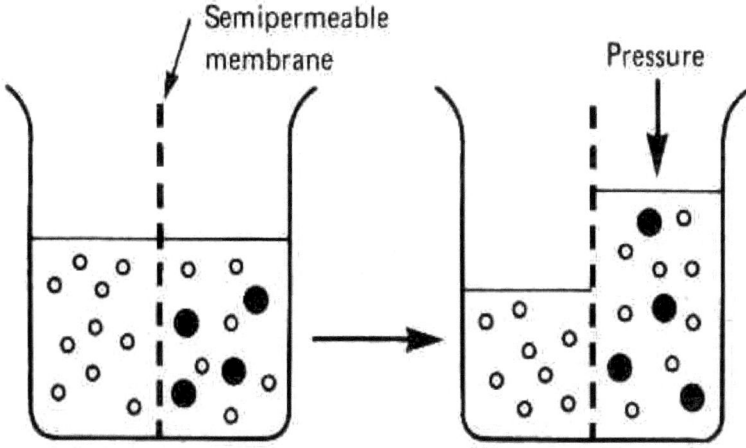

As it was said, some substances can freely pass through the cell membrane but others cannot. So, the cell recruits special mechanisms which we can divide them according to the use of energy. If, for the transport of a substance is not needed energy then we speak for passive transport which always occurs in the direction of the concentration gradient. When the cell uses energy for transport of substances it is said as active transport, it is against the concentration gradient (this is why it needs energy), and it is divided into pinocytosis, and phagocytosis.

Pinocytosis is a form of endocytosis in which small liquid particles are brought into the cell suspended within small vesicles which subsequently fuse with lysosomes to hydrolyze, or to break down, the particles.

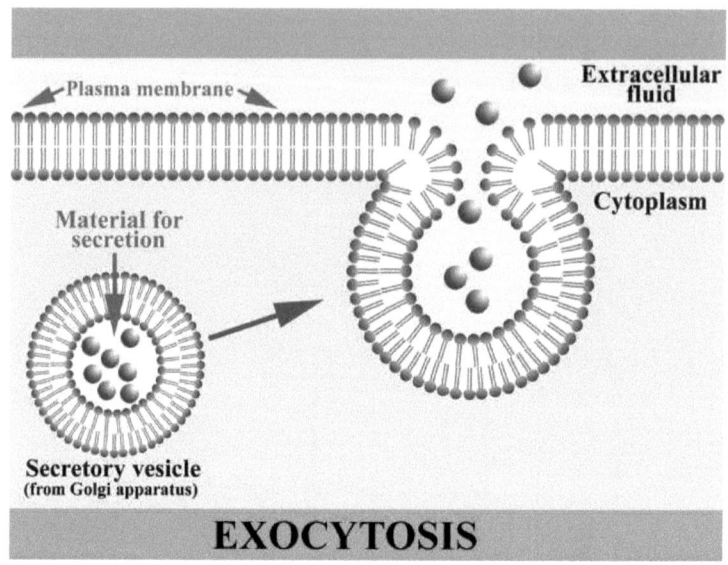

EXOCYTOSIS

Phagocytosis is a specific form of endocytosis involving the vesicular internalization of solid particles, such as bacteria. Phagocytosis is involved in the acquisition of nutrients from the environment, and in the immune system. For example, the macrophages through phagocytosis engulf bacteria. This phagocytotic vesicle will fuse with the primary lysosomes forming thus the secondary lysosomes. The enzymes of the lysosomes will finally kill the bacteria.

Exocytosis is a reverse way of transport than endocytosis. It is the process by which a cell directs the contents of secretory vesicles out of the cell membrane. These membrane-bound vesicles contain soluble proteins which are secreted to the extracellular environment, as well as membrane proteins and lipids that are sent to become components of the cell membrane. The proteins that are to be excreted are formed in the ribosomes of rough endoplasmic reticulum. Then they are transferred to Golgi apparatus for some modification, and then are excreted. This is the way, for example, that protein hormones are produced and excreted from the cell.

1.2) Cell organelles

The cell organelles are suspended in the gelatinous fluid of cytosol and are adapted and/or specialized for carrying out one or more vital functions.

Plastids are major organelles found in the cells of plants and are the site of manufacture and storage of important chemical compounds used by the cell. Plastids often contain pigments used in photosynthesis, and the types of pigments present, can change or determine the cell's colour. Plastids are responsible for photosynthesis (chloroplasts), storage of reserve substances, like starch.

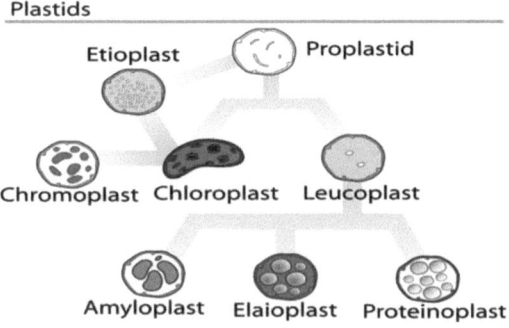

Thylakoids are membrane-bound compartments inside chloroplasts and cyanobacteria. They are the site of the light-dependent reactions of photosynthesis.

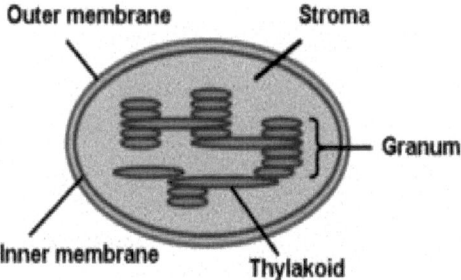

Ribosomes is a large complex of rRNA and protein molecules. They consist of two subunits, and act as an assembly line where RNA from the nucleus is used to synthesize

11

proteins from amino acids. Ribosomes can be found either floating freely or bound to a membrane (the rough endoplasmatic reticulum in eukaryotes, or the cell membrane in prokaryotes). Prokaryotes have 70S (Svedberg) ribosomes, each consisting of a small (30S) and a large (50S) subunit. Svedberg unit, is a measure of the rate of sedimentation in centrifugation, rather than size and accounts for why fragment names do not add up (70S is made of 50S and 30S). Eukaryotes have 80S ribosomes, each consisting of a small (40S) and large (60S) subunit. Free ribosomes, which are floating to the cytosol, are producing proteins that will stay inside the cell and will be used as functional and structural components. The membrane bound ribosomes synthesize proteins that are going to be expelled from the cell (through exocytosis) and will be used in a distance from them e.g. protein hormones.

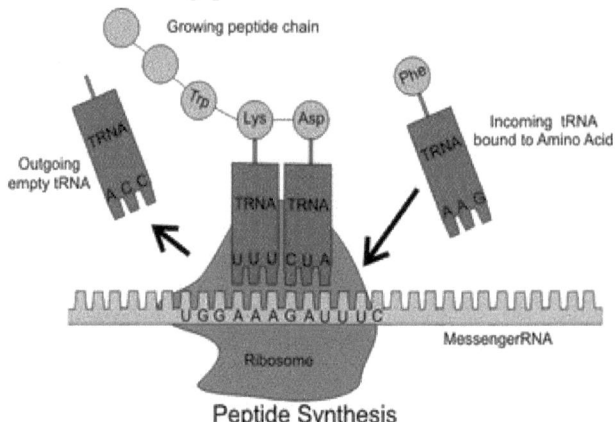

Peptide Synthesis

Mitochondria are self-replicating organelles that occur in various numbers, shapes, and sizes in the cytoplasm of all eukaryotic cells. Mitochondria play a critical role in generation of energy in the eukaryotic cell (Krebs cycle is located inside mitochondria). Mitochondria contain their own DNA or RNA which is different from the nuclear, and it is much like that of prokaryotic cells, strongly supporting thus the evolutionary theory of endosymbiosis, according to which mitochondria where free organisms in the past, that were trapped inside the cell of eukaryotes and in this form appear today. Mitochondria have 99% heredity from the mother to the child. That highlights that our metabolic pathways are majorly influenced from the metabolism of our mothers.

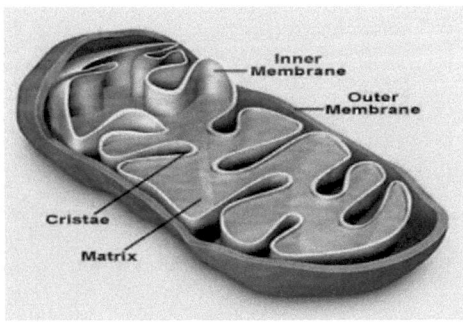

Lysosomes contain digestive enzymes (proteases, saccharases, hydrolases, lipases) and digest excess or worn-out organelles, food particles, and engulfed viruses or bacteria. The cell could not house these destructive enzymes if they were not contained in a membrane-bound system.

Lysosome Structure

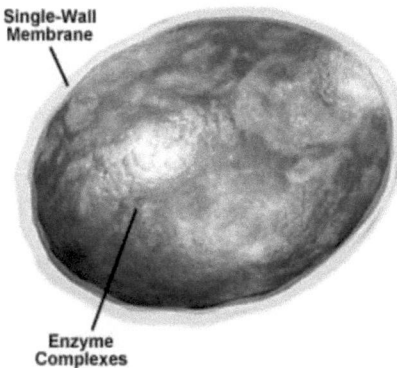

Endoplasmic reticulum forms an interconnected network of tubules, vesicles, and cisternae within cells. We can divide it into smooth endoplasmic reticulum, and rough endoplasmic reticulum. Smooth endoplasmic reticulum (lucks ribosomes) synthesize lipids and steroids, metabolize carbohydrates and steroids, and regulate calcium concentration, drug detoxification, and attachment of receptors on cell membrane proteins. Rough endoplasmic reticulum has its membranes covered with ribosomes from where it owns its name. In an electron microscope section it appears rough due to the presence of ribosomes. Proteins that are synthesized in rough endoplasmic reticulum they are then transferred to the Golgi apparatus for posttranslational modifications. Then from the Golgi apparatus they are expelled from the cell.

Endoplasmic Reticulum

Smooth Endoplasmic Reticulum

Nuclear Pore

Nuclear Envelope

Cisternal Space

Rough Endoplasmic Reticulum

Cisternae

Ribosomes

Golgi apparatus was discovered by the Italian physician Camillo Golgi in 1898. The primary function of Golgi apparatus is to receive proteins and lipids (cis-face), synthesized in endoplasmic reticulum. Inside the membranous sacs of the apparatus there is an adjustment and modification of the received substances, after which they packaged in vesicles for secretion from the cell (trans-face).

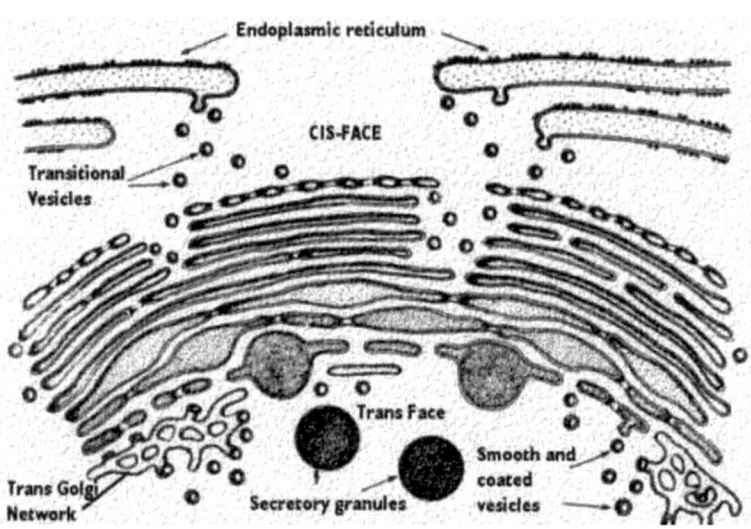

Endoplasmic reticulum

CIS-FACE

Transitional Vesicles

Trans Face

Trans Golgi Network

Secretory granules

Smooth and coated vesicles

Nucleus possesses a central role in the life of the cell. It is the place where the genetic material, in a form of DNA and RNA, is kept and gives the appropriate instructions for all the functions of cell. It can be single, or in multiple copies and it can posses a central or peripheral position in the cell. The nucleus is separated from the cytoplasm by a double membrane called the nuclear envelope. The nuclear envelope has pores so as to

14

communicate with the cytoplasm. Nucleolus is a non-membrane bound structure, found within nucleus, and is responsible for the production of rRNA (structural component of ribosomes).

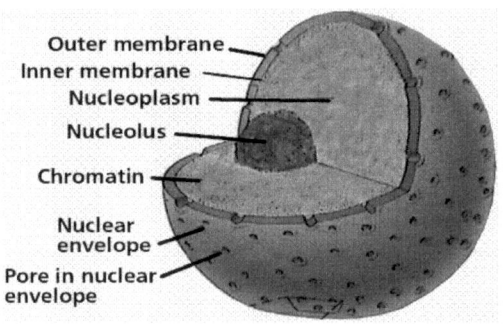

1.3) Cell division

Cell division is the process by which a single cell (mother cell) is dividing into two daughter cells that contain qualitative and quantitative the same amount of genetic material.

Prokaryotes divide by binary fission, a process much more simple than the division of eukaryotes, which gives rise to identical cells without any sign of cell differentiation.

Eukaryotes divide in a more complicate way which is comprised of karyokinesis (mitosis, or meiosis), and cytokinesis.

The cell life cycle comprises the following stages: G1 phase, S phase, G2 phase, mitosis. Mitosis incorporates prophase, metaphase, anaphase, and telophase. After these phases follows cytokinesis.

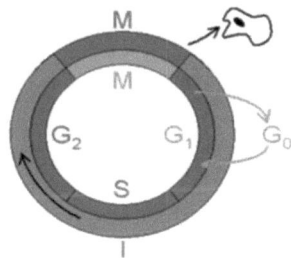

G o phase exists in cells that have exit the cell cycle temporarily with the ability to reenter to cycle after demand e.g. stem cells, or have permanently exit the cycle e.g. neurons (they don't have the ability to divide).

G_1 phase is a period in the cell cycle during interphase, before the S phase. For many cells, this phase is the major period of cell growth during their lifespan. During this stage new organelles are being synthesized, so the cell requires both structural proteins and enzymes, resulting in great amount of protein synthesis and a high metabolic rate in the cell.

S phase (Synthesis) is a period in the cell cycle during interphase, between G_1 phase and the G_2 phase. Following G_1, the cell enters the S stage, where DNA synthesis or replication occurs. At the beginning of the S stage, each chromosome is composed of one coiled DNA double helix molecule, which is called a chromatid. At the end of this stage, each chromosome has two identical DNA double helix molecules, and therefore is composed of two sister chromatids (joined at the centromere). The end result is the existence of duplicated genetic material in the cell, which will eventually be divided into two.

G_2 phase is the third, final, and usually the shortest phase during interphase within the cell cycle, in which the cell undergoes a period of rapid growth to prepare for mitosis. It follows successful completion of DNA synthesis and chromosomal replication during the S phase.

At the end of these stages, follows mitosis:

Prophase is the process by which loosely coiled chromatin inside nucleus, condenses together into a highly ordered structure called a chromosome. Since the genetic material has already been duplicated earlier in S phase, the replicated chromosomes have two sister chromatids, bound together at the centromere.

Metaphase is the process by which the centromeres of the chromosomes convene along the metaphase plate or equatorial plane, an imaginary line that is in equal distant from the two centrosome poles.

Anaphase is the process by which the sister chromatids which have become distinct sister chromosomes, are pulled apart and move toward the respective centrosomes to which they are attached. Next the centrosomes move apart to the opposite poles of the cell.

Telophase is the process by which sister chromosomes attach at opposite ends of the cell. A new nuclear envelope, using fragments of the parent cell's nuclear membrane, forms around each set of separated sister chromosomes. Both sets of chromosomes, now surrounded by new nuclei, unfold back into chromatin.

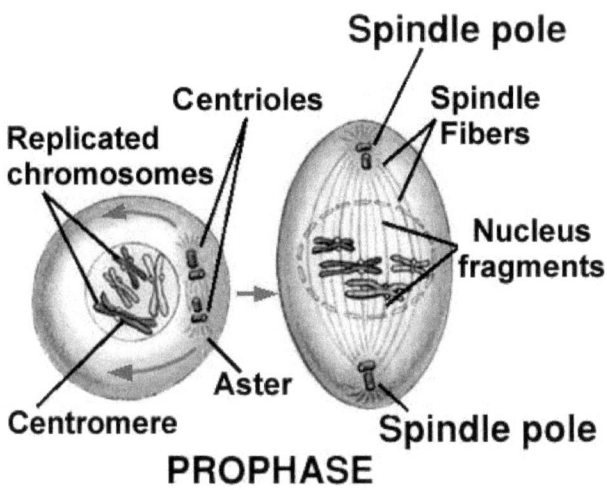

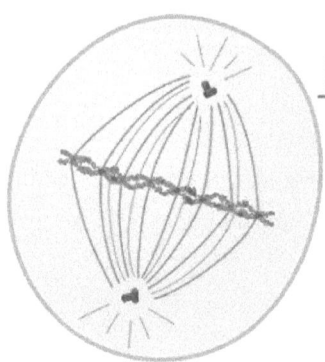

Metaphase

Chromosomes line up
along **metaphase plate**
(imaginary plane)

Anaphase

Chromosomes break at
centromeres, and **sister
chromatids** move to opposite
ends of the cell

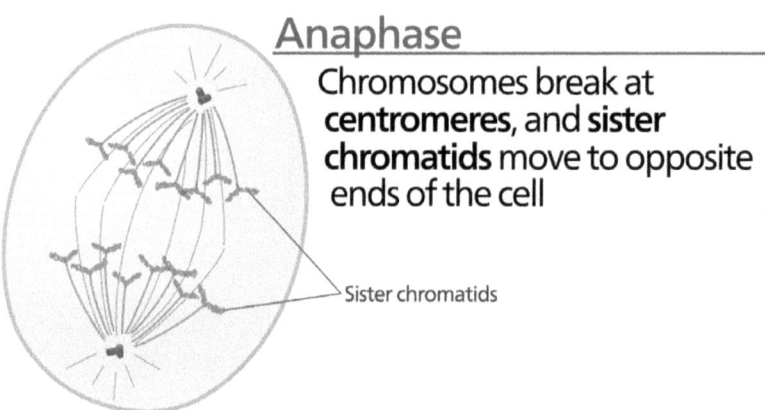

Sister chromatids

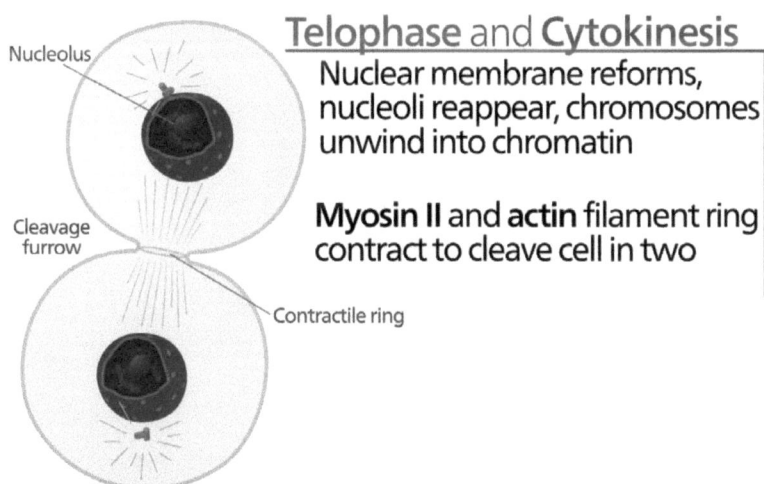

Nucleolus

Cleavage
furrow

Contractile ring

Telophase and Cytokinesis
Nuclear membrane reforms,
nucleoli reappear, chromosomes
unwind into chromatin

Myosin II and **actin** filament ring
contract to cleave cell in two

Meiosis divides diploid cells and through two successive reductive divisions produces four haploid cells which are called gametes. So, by this way the ovum has an haploid germ line, and the spermatozoon also has an haploid germ line. When the spermatozoon fertilizes the ovum we have the production of a diploid zygote, which will then divide mitoticaly to give rise to the embryo through a series of cell proliferations and differentiations.

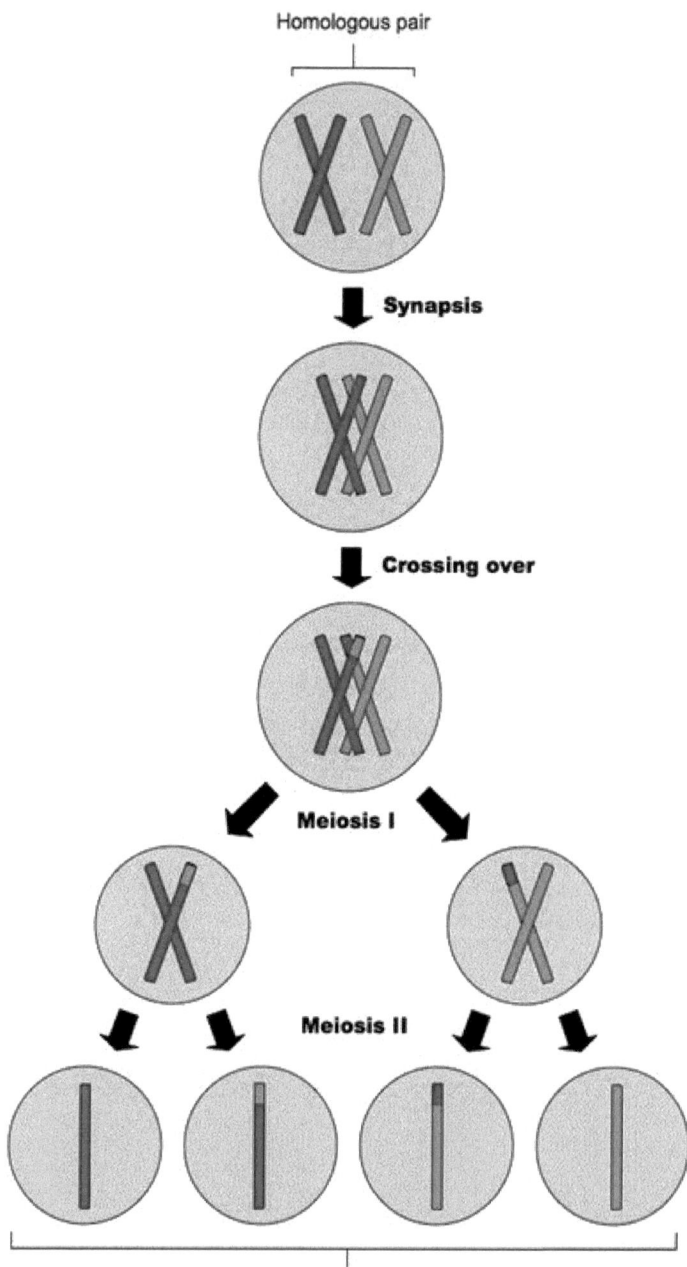

Homologous pair

Synapsis

Crossing over

Meiosis I

Meiosis II

Four genetically distinct haploid daughter cells
(middle two are *recombinants*)

2) The plant

Plants are eukaryotic living organisms with a variable size ranging from single cell organisms, to multicellular organisms.

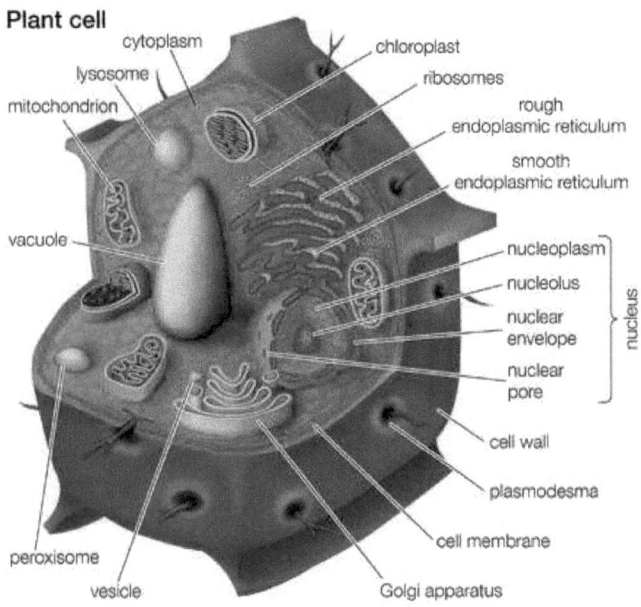

According to their mode of nutrition, we can list them in the following groups:

A mixotrophic plant can use for its nutrition a mix of different sources of energy. They can combine autotrophic and heterotrophic mechanisms for obtain the necessary elements for survival.

An autotrophic plant can produce complex organic compounds from simple inorganic molecules by using the energy of light (through photosynthesis), or through inorganic chemical reactions (chemosynthesis).

An heterotrophic plant obtains energy from light, but needs carbon in an organic form for growth.

A saprophytic plant through mineralization of organic substances found in the soil, processes the dead organic matter, and thus participates in the cycle of substances.

Carnivorous plants are plants that derive some or most of their nutrients from trapping and consuming animals or protozoans, typically insects and other arthropods. In this way they adapt to grow in places where the soil is thin or poor in nutrients, especially nitrogen.

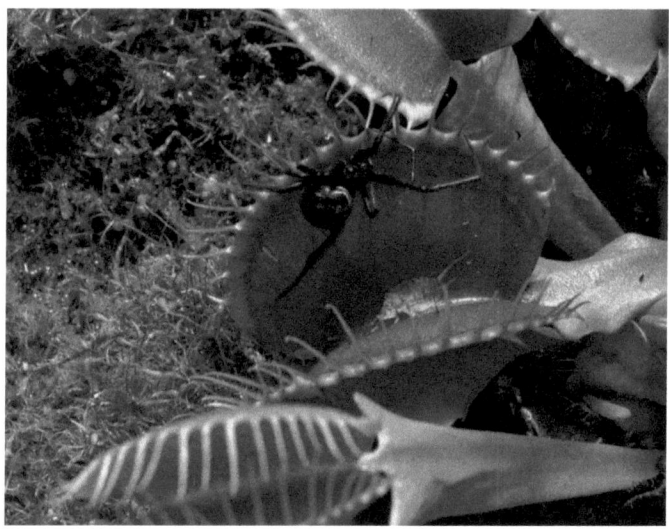

2.1) The leaf

Leaf is an above-ground plant organ specialized for photosynthesis through its chloroplasts. For this purpose, a leaf is typically flat (laminar) and thin. Leaves are also the sites in most plants where transpiration and storage of food and water occurs. It is composed of a lamina and the petiole (stalk). According to morphology we can distinguish a simple leaf which has only one lamina per leaf, and the compound leaf which has many distinct laminae per leaf. According to structure we can divide them into monofacial and bifacial leaves. The mesophyll of monofacial leaves doesn't show any signs of differentiation. In the contrary the parenchyma of bifacial leaves it is well organized into palisade and sponge parenchyma.

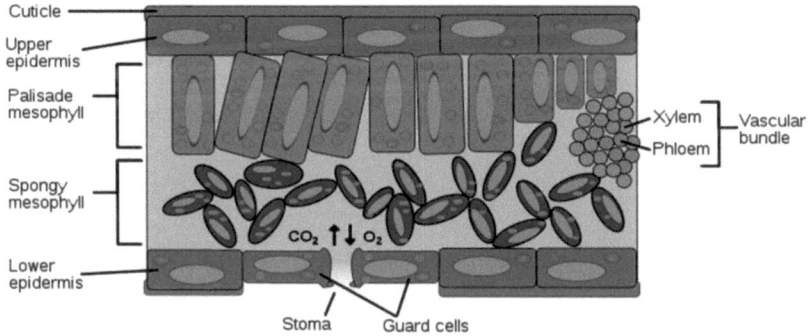

Epidermis is the outer layer of cells covering the leaf. It is usually transparent and covered from the outside with a waxy cuticle that prevents water loss and protects from insects. The epidermis tissue includes several differentiated cell types: epidermal cells, guard cells and epidermal hairs (trichomes). The guard cells surround the stomata and control the water evaporation and exchange of gases. Trichomes can be covering, stinging, and absorptive according to their function.

2.2) Venation of the leaf

It is the arrangement of the veins (xylem and phloem) that can be seen on the surface of a leaf. These veins belong to the general vascular bundle of the plant. We can distinguish three main types: parallel, pinnate, and palmate.

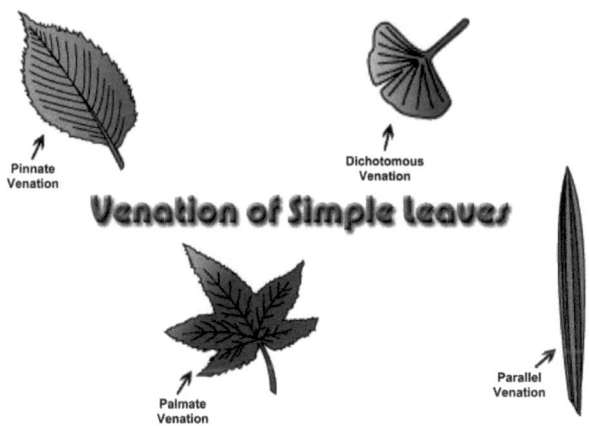

2.3) Inflorescence

Inflorescence is a group or cluster of flowers arranged on a stem that is composed of a main branch or a complicated arrangement of branches. The stem holding the whole inflorescence is called a peduncle, and the main stem holding the flowers or more branches within the inflorescence is called the rachis. The stalk of each single flower is called a pedicel. Inflorescences according to their mode of branching can be classified into simple or compound.

Simple inflorescences are classified into indeterminate, and determinate. Indeterminate simple inflorescences are generally called racemose and can be further subdivided into: raceme, spike, corymb, umbel, spadix, and capitulum. A raceme is an unbranched, indeterminate inflorescence, with pedicellate (short floral stalks) flowers along the axis.

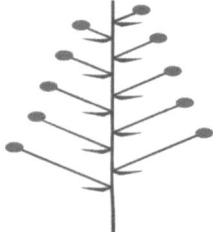

A spike is a type of raceme, with flowers that do not have a pedicel.

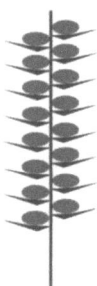

A corymb is an unbranched, indeterminate inflorescence that is flat-topped or convex due to their outer pedicels, which are progressively longer than inner ones.

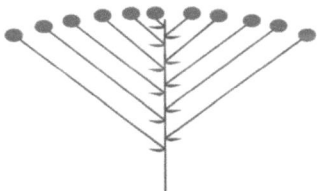

An umbel is a type of raceme with a short axis and multiple floral pedicels of equal length that appear to arise from a common point.

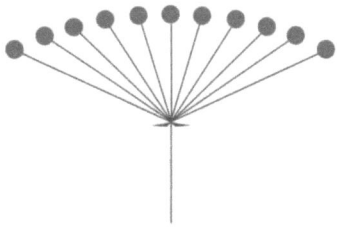

A spadix is a spike of flowers densely arranged around it, enclosed or accompanied by a highly specialized bract called a spathe.

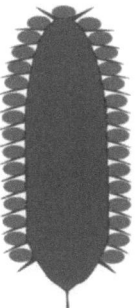

Capitulum is a very contracted raceme in which the single sessile flowers are borne on an enlarged stem.

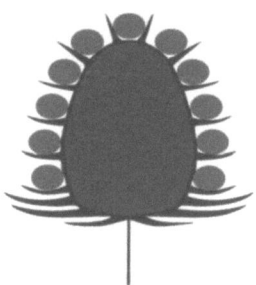

Determinate simple inflorescences are generally called cymose. The main type of cymose inflorescence is the cyme, which can be subdivided into bostryx (or helicoid cyme), drepanium, and scorpioid cyme.

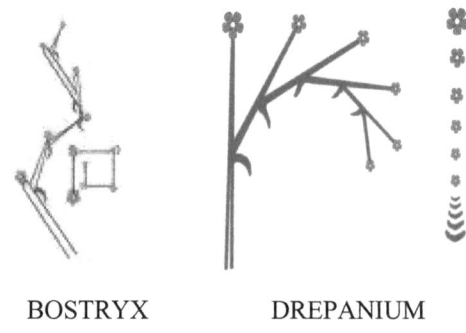

BOSTRYX   DREPANIUM

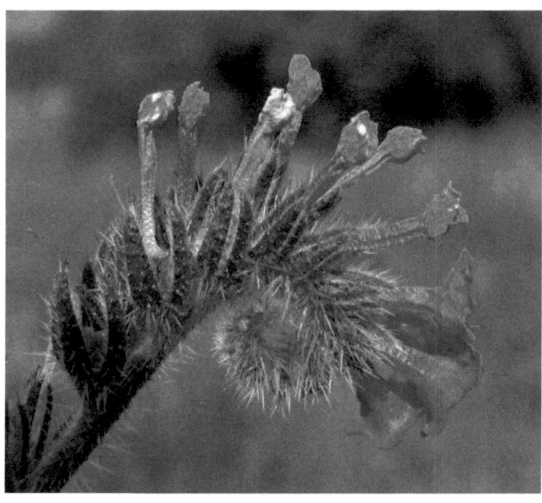

Scorpioid cyme

2.4) The seed

A seed is a small embryonic plant which is the product of gymnosperms and angiosperms, after fertilization of the flowers in the mother plant, through pollination. Seeds have an important role in the reproduction and spread of flowering plants, by means of several ways, such as the wind, water, or animals.

A typical seed includes three basic parts: (1) an embryo, (2) a supply of nutrients for the embryo, and (3) a seed coat.

The embryo is an immature plant from which a new plant will grow under proper conditions. The embryo has one cotyledon in the monocotyledons, and two cotyledons in the dicotyledons. The radicle is the embryonic root. The embryonic stem below the point of attachment of the cotyledon(s) is the hypocotyl. The hypocotyl is the primary organ of extension of the young plant and develops into the stem.

Within the seed, there is usually a store of nutrients for the nourishment of the developing embryo. The form of the stored nutrition varies depending on the kind of plant. In angiosperms, the stored food begins as a tissue called the endosperm, which is derived from the parent plant via double fertilization (typical for Magnoliophyta). This will result in the production of a triploid endosperm, rich in oil, or starch and proteins, and a diploid perisperm.

The seed coat (or testa) surrounds the developing embryo so as to protect it from dehydration and mechanical injury. It can be a paper-thin layer, or more hard and thick such as on coconut.

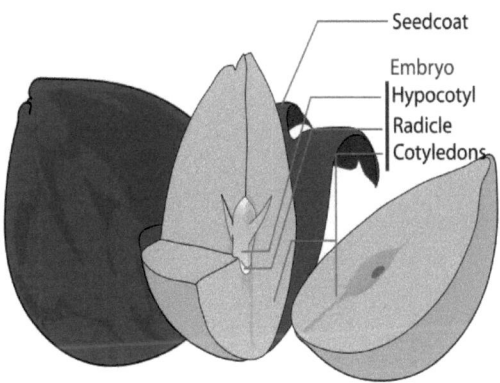

Seedcoat

Embryo
Hypocotyl
Radicle
Cotyledons

2.5) Vascular bundle of the plant

Each plant needs water and inorganic substances for its survival and reproduction. It needs a way so as these absorbed substances from the soil can be sufficiently move to the places where photosynthesis takes place, the leaves. It is remarkable that trees with many meters high can support that movement through diapnoe. That conductive system, from the root up to the leaves, consist the vascular bundle of the plants, and is represented through the veins. The veins are made up of xylem and phloem. Xylem brings water and minerals from the roots to the leaves. This is made when water potential of the root cells is more negative than that of the soil, usually due to high concentrations of solute, and water can move by osmosis into the root from the soil. This causes a positive pressure that forces water and minerals up the xylem towards the leaves. The phloem carries the products of photosynthesis from the leaves to every part of the plant where are needed. These are organic nutrients, particularly sucrose.

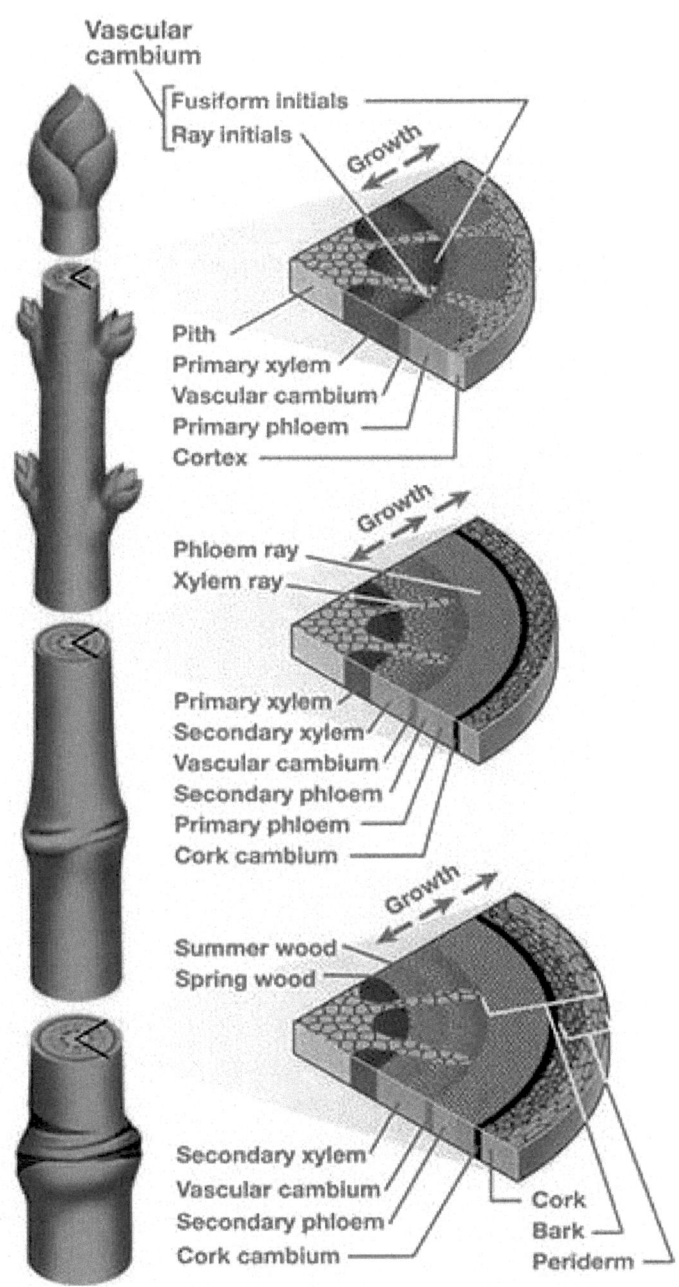

2.6) The root

Root is the organ of a plant that typically lies below the surface of the soil. The three major functions of roots are 1) absorption of water and inorganic nutrients, 2) anchoring of the plant body to the ground and 3) storage of food and nutrients. The roots can be classified into: aerial, prop, reserve, symbiotic, and Haustoria roots.

Aerial roots are entirely above the ground and they function as prop roots. They are found in areas with stagnated water.

Reserve roots are modified for storage of food or water e.g. in carrots.

Symbiotic roots are found in plants which enter into symbiosis with certain fungi to form mycorrhizas, and a large range of other organisms including bacteria. In this mutualistic association the plant provides the microorganisms with carbohydrates, and the microbes provide to the plant with phosphate ions and nitrogen, which the plant cannot obtain on its own.

Haustoria roots are called the roots of parasitic plants, which can absorb water and nutrients from an other plant.

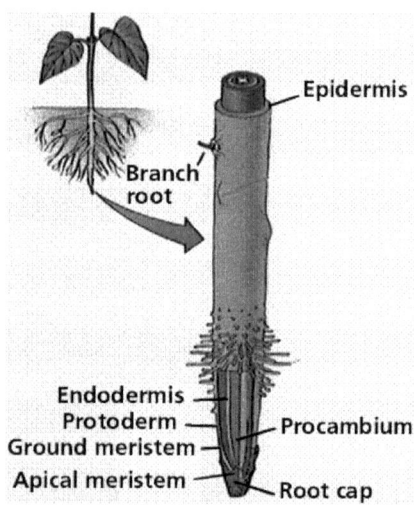

3) Genetics

Genetics made its first steps in the mid-1800s with the applied and theoretical research of Gregor Mendel. Nowadays it is a highly evolutionary science with a range of appliances in the modern Biology and Medicine. Genetics is the study of gene structure, function, and transmission of hereditary signs from parents to children. These hereditary signs are encoded in genes which are the main keepers of genetic information.

3.1) Genes

A gene is a sequence of nucleic acid (DNA, or in case of some viruses RNA) which provides the information for the coding of an RNA, or protein, necessary for the organism. The combination of all genes in an organism is called genotype, or genome. Each organism has multiple copies of genes which encode for a same characteristic but in a different mode, these are called alleles. For example, human genome has many alleles which determine the color of the eye. All alleles control the same characteristic (color), but in a different way (brown, blue, or green eyes). Alleles can be classified as dominant, and recessive. Dominant are those who under certain environmental circumstances give a phenotypic sign, either in an homozygous or heterozygous combination. Recessive alleles must be in homozygous combination so as to give phenotypic manifestation.

As it said before, genes control every part and manifestation of our life: from our external appearance, biochemical pathways, enzymatic functions, to our psychology. Thus, it is important to exist a sufficient level of regulatory mechanisms which will control when the genes will be expressed, for how much time, and that the organism will obtain the necessary amount of product. All genes have regulatory regions for that purpose. A regulatory region shared by almost all genes is known as the promoter, which provides a position that is recognized by the transcription machinery, when a gene is about to be transcribed and expressed. A gene can have more than one promoter, resulting in RNAs that differ in how far they extend in the 5' end (transcription has 5 to 3 direction). Some genes have "strong" promoters that bind the transcription machinery well, and others have "weak" promoters that bind it poorly. These "weak" promoters usually permit a lower rate of transcription than the "strong" promoters, because the transcription machinery binds to them and initiates transcription less frequently. An other possible regulatory region include enhancers, which can be bound with proteins (transcription factors), so as to enhance the transcription rate of the gene they control. Most regulatory regions are located upstream-towards the 5 end of the nucleic acid sequence. Eukaryotic promoter regions are much more complex and difficult to identify than prokaryotic promoters.

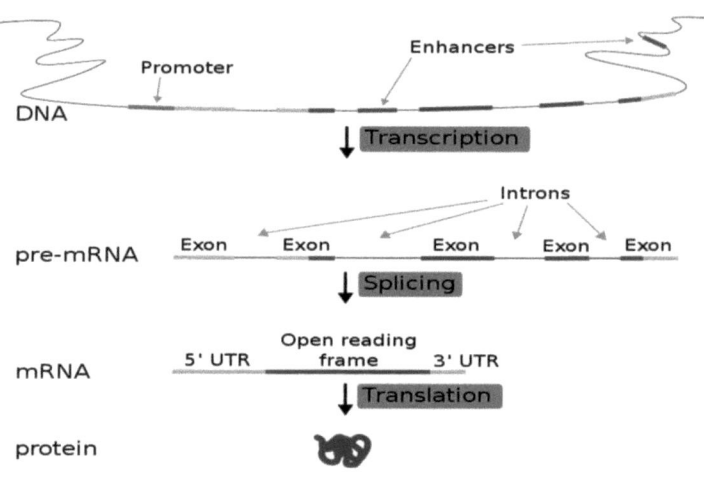

Many prokaryotic genes are organized into operons, which are group of genes that are transcribed as a unit, and are controlled by the same regulatory regions. This is in contrast with the eukaryotic organisms, where every gene has its own regulatory region. This also highlights the grater complexity of the eukaryotes in comparison with prokaryotes. Prokaryotes may also have additional genetic information located on plasmids. Plasmids contain little amount of genes which usually concern resistance to some antibiotics. These plasmids can be transferred from one bacterium to an other, through conjugation, giving thus to other bacteria the ability of being resistant to some antibiotics.

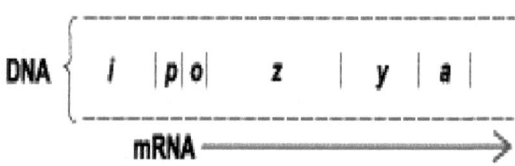

3.2) Chromosomes

The total complement of genes in a cell (genome) may be stored on one or more chromosomes. The region of the chromosome at which a particular gene is located is called locus. A chromosome consists of a single, very long DNA helix on which thousands of genes may be found. It is well known today that each chromosome does not contain the same amount of genes in all of its length. So, there are genetic deserts in which no gene can be found, and other regions that are rich in genes. Every human somatic (diploid) cell contains 44 autosomes (half from the mother, and half from the father), and 2 sexual chromosomes or gonosomes (X, Y) giving thus a net number of 46 chromosomes. The total number of chromosomes, which is characteristic for every animal species, is called karyotype. Chromosomes are organized in the human karyotype into seven groups: group A (1-3), group B (4-5), group C (6-12), group D (13-15), group E (16-18), group F (19-20), group G (21-22).

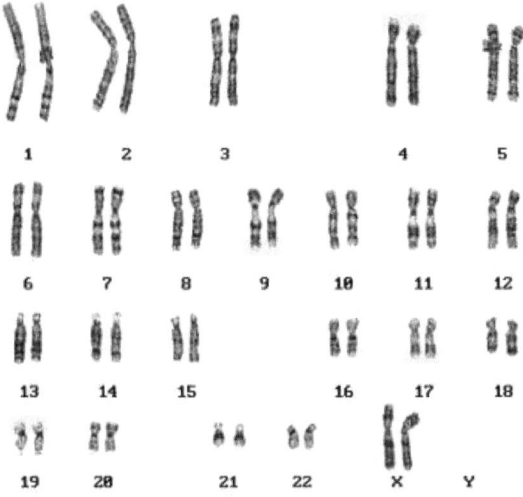

As it was mentioned, every human somatic cell has the same number of chromosomes, thereby the same genes. But in every cell there is a different part of DNA that is being expressed, so different products produced, so finally different organs and tissues.

The gene expression is a dynamic correlation between genotype, environment, and phenotype. For example, there is a family with the father's height 183 cm, mother's height 175 cm and the child's height 190 cm. That indicates that the child has in its genome the information for a range of height e.g. up until 195 cm. Under the given environmental conditions the child will have the minimum of height when for example it doesn't have sufficient supply of nutrients, or he will get the maximum possible height (195 cm) when he grows in optimum environmental conditions e.g. sufficient supply of nutrients.

3.3) Mutations

Mutations are changes in the DNA sequence of a cell's genome, which can result in the alteration of the gene product, and prevent the gene from functioning properly or completely loss of its function. Some mutations may have no effect on the gene product (silent mutations). Those who do affect the gene product may lead to the production of a protein which is not functioning correctly, or is produced in fewer amounts than needed. In the case that mutation affects the production of an enzyme, it may have detrimental consequences on the metabolism of the individual. Mutations can be classified as spontaneous and induced. Spontaneous mutations may occur in nature without the involvement of the human e.g. due to sun irradiation. Induced mutations occur in the laboratory by the man, e.g. to put in the DNA, base analogues to see how the DNA will react and if it will be still functioning.

We can also classify mutations 1) according to their effect on structure e.g. chromosomal mutations, which affect the structure of chromosomes, 2) according to their effect on function e.g. when there is loss of function of the gene, or gain of function in a previously non coding gene, and 3) according to their effect on fitness e.g. harmful mutation (decreases the fitness of the organism), beneficial mutation (increases the fitness of the organism), neutral mutation (has no harmful or beneficial effect on the organism).

Every mutation, independently of its source, is under the pressure of natural selection. Thus, if the organism after mutation obtains characteristics that will allow him to survive better in his environment, he will pass these advantageous new genes to the next generations. If after the mutation are produced genes that make the survival of the organism more difficult, that organism will eventually die, so these genes will not pass to the next generations.

Genes mutations is a way through which evolution and natural selection produced all that great range of genes that exist today. The primitive organisms didn't have such a great amount of genes. After mutations there where produced new genes from which only the advantageous where surviving. With the passage of years new mutations where accumulating and only the advantageous where passing to the next generations. This process was repeated again and again leading thus to the today's great variability.

3.4) Replication

DNA replication is a fundamental process occurring in all living organisms so as to copy their DNA. At the end of this process the daughter cells must have quantitative and qualitative the same amount of DNA as the mother cell. In the cell DNA replication begins in the replication fork. There, is recruited an enzyme, the DNA helicase, which helps to untwist the twisted DNA helix, allowing thus the next enzymes of replication to approach. As the DNA helicase moves on, it leaves on its behind the two separated strands of DNA. One of them is the leading strand, and the other the lagging strand. The leading strand allows the synthesis of a continuous strand of DNA in direction 5' to 3'. For the initiation of synthesis is required a short segment of RNA (primer) which will then allow the DNA polymerase to elongate the chain. The DNA polymerase is uncapapable to initiate the replication without the RNA primer. This polymerase is a DNA polymerase III (DNA Pol III) in prokaryotes, and Pol ε in eukaryotes. It elongates the chain by adding new nucleotides to the 3' end and links them with phosphodiester bonds. The nucleotides are added according to the template with adenine (A) always combined with thymine (T), and guanine (G) always combined with cytosine (C). The lagging strand does not allow the synthesis of a continuous strand of DNA but the synthesis goes step by step through the Okazaki fragments. So, here we have the synthesis of multiple DNA segments (Okazaki fragments) which are then linked together to produce a continuous chain of DNA. Every segment needs an RNA primer so as the DNA polymerase can act (like in leading strand). DNA polymerase III or Pol δ lengthens the primer segments, forming thus the Okazaki fragments. Primer removal in eukaryotes is performed by Pol δ . At the end of the whole process of replication an enzyme, DNA ligase, connects the complementary strands together through hydrogen bonding.

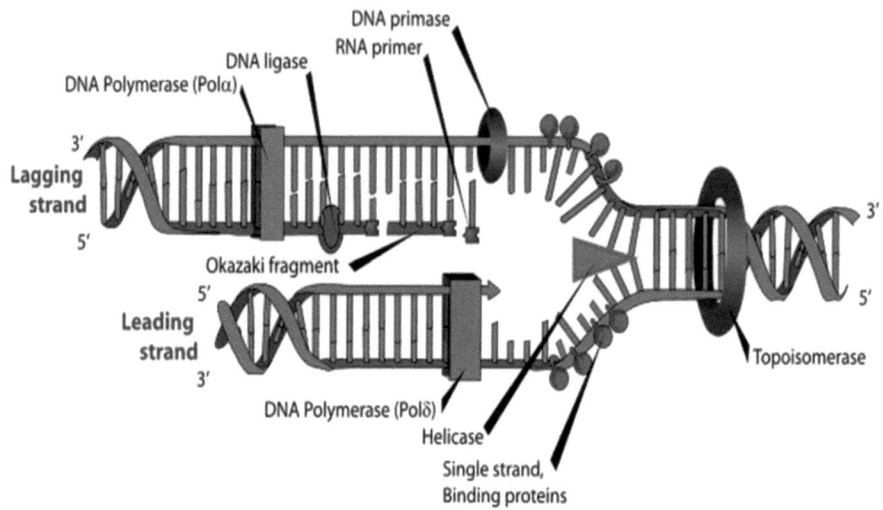

DNA primase
RNA primer
DNA ligase
DNA Polymerase (Polα)

3'
Lagging
strand
5'

Okazaki fragment

5'
Leading
strand
3'

DNA Polymerase (Polδ)
Helicase
Single strand,
Binding proteins

Topoisomerase

3'

5'

3.5) Transcription

Transcription is the process of RNA synthesis using as a template a strand of DNA. This occurs during the process of expression of the genetic information and can produce a range of RNA molecules: messenger RNA (mRNA), transfer RNA (tRNA), ribosomal RNA (rRNA), and small nuclear RNA (snRNA). Only the mRNA can continue, through translation, to the production of proteins. The stretch of DNA transcribed into an RNA molecule is called a transcription unit and includes at least one gene. Transcription has some control mechanisms, but they are fewer and less effective than the control of DNA replication; therefore, transcription has a lower copying fidelity than DNA replication. DNA transcription has a 5' to 3' direction, as DNA replication. Although DNA is arranged in two antiparallel strands, only one of the two DNA strands, called the template strand, is used for transcription. This is because the produced RNA is single stranded. The other DNA strand is called the coding strand, because its sequence is the same as the newly created RNA transcript (with the exception that RNA contains uracil instead of thymine). Transcription is divided into five stages: pre-initiation, initiation, promoter clearance, elongation and termination.

Pre-initiation is the process that precedes the binding of RNA polymerase which will permit the initiation of transcription. In eukaryotes, RNA polymerase requires for its binding the presence of a core promoter sequence in the DNA. Core promoters are sequences within the promoter region of DNA which are essential for initiation of transcription. They are located upstream from the start site of transcription. RNA polymerase is able to bind to core promoters in the presence of various specific transcription factors. The most common type of core promoter in eukaryotes is a short DNA sequence known as TATA box. The TATA box is the binding site for a range of transcription factors which will eventually allow to the RNA polymerase to approach. Other proteins, such as activators (which increase the transcription rate), and repressors (which decrease the transcription rate) are used to modulate the transcription rate, according to the needs of the cell.

Initiation is the process in which RNA polymerase approaches after all the DNA segment which is to be transcribed, with the aid of transcription factors. The binding of RNA polymerase signals the initiation of transcription. The completed assembly of transcription factors and RNA polymerase bind to the promoter are forming the transcription initiation complex. In the whole length of the DNA strand there may be found at the same time a lot of transcription initiation complexes, which transcript different segments of DNA.

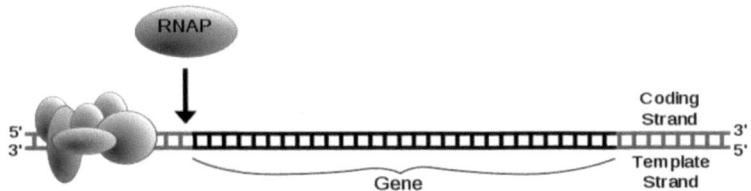

Promoter clearance is the process in which RNA polymerase moves from the promoter region allowing thus an other RNA polymerase to approach and start again the transcription (when a lot of RNA polymerases are transcribing at the same time, the same segment of DNA this is called a polysome). This is a critical step until RNA polymerase can produce a transcript of 23 nucleotides. Before that number of nucleotides is reached, RNA polymerase can lead to abortive transcriptions, which are released transcripts with a length of less than 23 nucleotides, with no function. Once the critical number of the 23 nucleotides is reached, then the RNA polymerase does no longer slips, and the elongation can occur.

Elongation is the process through which RNA polymerase moves on the template strand and uses base pairing, complementary with the DNA template to create an RNA copy. That produces an RNA molecule which is an exact copy of the coding strand (with uracil instead of thymine, and riboses, instead of DNA deoxyriboses).

Coding strand   ATGCATGC
Template strand   TACGTACG
RNA molecule   AUGCAUGC

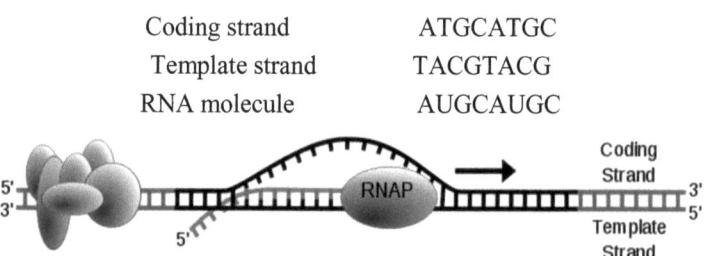

Termination signals the termination of the transcription process, cleavage and release of the new RNA transcript.

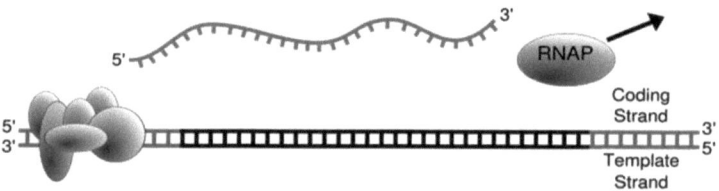

3.6) Translation

Translation is the final step of gene expression and leads to the production of proteins. The special case of translation concerns that the "language" of nucleotides must be translated to a different "language" of amino acids. So, we have two different "languages" which need to find a common way, so as to understand its other. This common way is given through the genetic code. The genetic code can be said, in simple terms, that is a vocabulary which translates the "language" of nucleotides, to the "language" of amino acids. The nucleotides which are to be translated are arranged in a particular way. For example the mRNA strand has the following nucleotides: AUGACGGCCUGA. These are read by the genetic code as three letter words: AUG/ACG/GCC/UGA and are translated to the twenty letter alphabet of amino acids. For the process of translation to occur is needed the mRNA which will act as a template, ribosomes (which are composed of rRNA and proteins), and tRNA which will bring the amino acids to the ribosomes. During the activation of amino acids, they are bound to one arm of the tRNA. The other arm bears the anticodon region which matches with the codon region of the mRNA. The codon region of the mRNA bears the three letter words of nucleotides, which are called codons.

4) Human Biology

The human body consists of approximately 220 different types of cells which are organized into several tissues, and organs (functional grouping of multiple tissues). In the following sections several tissues, organs, and organ systems found in the human body will be presented.

4.1) Bones

Bones form the skeleton of the human body and they are a type of dense connective tissue. Their function is to move, support, and protect the various organs. They also produce blood elements and store minerals. Other types of tissue found in bones include marrow, endosteum and periosteum, nerves, blood vessels and cartilage.

4.2) Vertebral column

The vertebral column (backbone or spine) is a column which usually consists of 33-34 vertebrae and is separated into five segments: cervical, thoracic, lumbar, sacral, and coccyx. It houses in its spinal canal, the spinal cord (part of the central nervous system). Between adjacent vertebrae are found the intervertebral discs which allow slight movements of the vertebrae and at the same time act as ligaments which hold the vertebrae together.

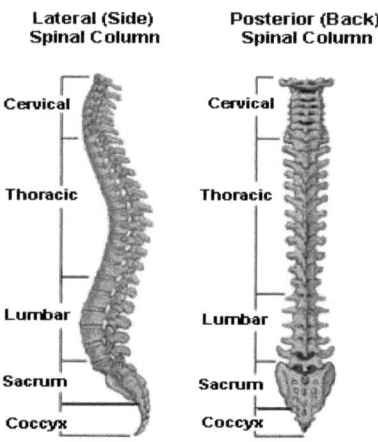

4.3) Muscles

The human body consists of approximately 600 muscles which according to their mode of innervation and structure, can be divided into three groups: striated, smooth, and cardiac.

Striated muscles are also called skeletal muscles highlightened thus their role in moving the skeleton of the body. Their control is under the influence of the somatic nervous system, thus they are subjected to our will. They consist of three parts: the origin, which attaches to the less movable part of the skeleton, the belly, and the insertion which ends to the more movable part of the skeleton. Skeletal muscle is made up from the aggregation of individual cells, known as muscle fibers. These cells (muscle fibers) are cylindrical, multinucleated and composed of actin-myosin myofibrils. The myofibrils are organized in a repeated manner, the sarcomeres, and are responsible for the contraction of the muscle cell, and the microscopic cross striated appearance of the muscle.

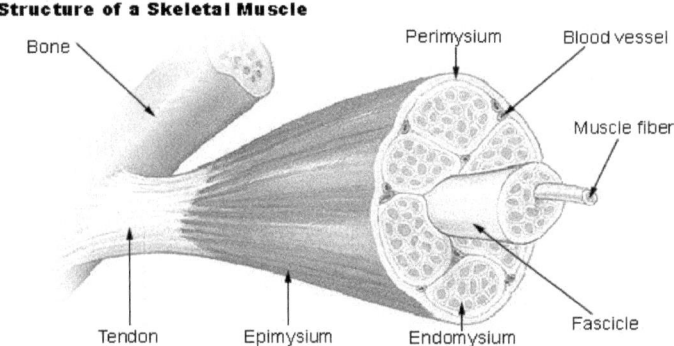

Smooth muscles are also called involuntary muscles. They are mostly found in the internal organs, and in the wall of blood vessels. They are called smooth because there is no cross striation seen in the microscope. They are under the influence of the autonomic nervous system; thereby they are not subjected to our will. Compared to the striated muscles, smooth muscles contract in a slower way e.g. peristaltic movements of the bowel, for a longer period of time, and they can be influenced by hormones e.g. stress hormones (adrenaline, noradrenaline) cause dilatation of the pupil of the eye.

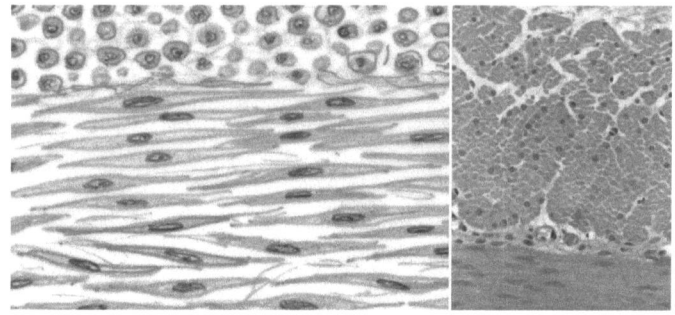

Cardiac muscle is found only in the hurt and has both characteristics of striated and smooth muscle: it has a microscopic cross striated appearance, but it is under the control of the autonomic nervous system.

4.4) Blood (composition and function)

Blood is an important body fluid which participates in a range of functions such as: thermoregulation of the body, acid- base (pH) regulation, transports to the cells oxygen and nutrients, and takes away from them the waste products of their metabolism. It is composed of blood cells and blood plasma. The blood cells found can be divided into red blood cells, white blood cells, and platelets. The plasma accounts for the 55% of the total blood volume and is composed of proteins, electrolytes, nutrients, waste products of metabolism of tissues, and the blood cells suspended into it.

Red blood cells have a characteristic shape of biconcave disc and during their maturity they lack nucleus and organelles. They contain hemoglobin which is an iron containing protein, responsible for the transport of oxygen to the tissues. That makes clear why a diet free of iron can lead to metabolic disturbances e.g. anemia. The proportion of blood occupied by red blood cells is referred to as the hematocrit, and it can increase in situations of lack of oxygen such as in a low atmospheric pressure of a high altitude.

White blood cells (leukocytes) are recruited when the body is triggering an immune response to defend its shelf against invading microorganisms. They divided into granulocytes (neutrophils, basophils, eosinophils), and agranulocytes (lymphocytes, monocytes, macrophages).

Neutrophils, are the most abundant type of white blood cells in human, and form an essential part of the innate immune system.

Basophils are the least common type of granulocytes. They store histamine, which can cause allergic reaction when secreted from the cells. Like all circulating granulocytes, basophils can be recruited out of the blood into a tissue when needed, through diapedesis.

Eosinophils account for 1-6% of white blood cells and are responsible for combating multicellular parasites. They contain histamine, which may lead to allergic reactions when secreted.

Lymphocytes are divided into natural-killer cells, B lymphocytes and T lymphocytes. Natural-killer cells defend the human body from tumors and virally infected cells. T and B lymphocytes are the major components of the adaptive (specific) immune response. B lymphocytes are responsible for the humoral immunity by the production of antibodies. They can also be used in the active immunization, when there is urgent need of antibodies and the organism has not the time to produce them on its own, and so we inject them to the high risk person. T lymphocytes produce cytokines (T helper cells), and cytotoxic substances (cytotoxic T cells). Both B and T lymphocytes after their activation produce also memory cells. Memory cells remain in the peripheral tissues and circulation for an extended period of time, ready to respond to the same antigen upon future exposure. So, in a following exposure there is a more quick activation, and thus response of the lymphocytes.

Monocytes have two main functions in the immune system: (1) replenish resident macrophages and dendritic cells and (2) in response to inflammation signals, monocytes can move quickly (approx. 8-12 hours) to sites of infection in the tissues and divide/differentiate into macrophages and dendritic cells to elicit an immune response.

Macrophages are produced by the differentiation of monocytes. Monocytes and macrophages are phagocytes, acting in both, non-specific defense (innate immunity) as well as to help initiate specific defense mechanisms (adaptive immunity).

Platelets or thrombocytes are cell fragments which are derived from megakaryocytes. They play a fundamental role in the formation of blood clots and production of growth factor so as to prevent bleeding and to promote healing.

4.5) Blood groups

Every individual has its own blood type which must be taken into account in several medical procedures such as transfusion. There are currently recognized at least 30 blood group systems, but the most frequently used are the ABO and Rhesus system. The classification is based on the antigens that are found on the surface of red blood cells.

BLOOD GROUP	ANTIGENS	ANTIBODIES
A	A	anti-B
B	B	anti-A
O	none	anti-B and anti-A

The Rhesus (Rh) blood group system currently consists of 50 defined blood group antigens among which the 5 antigens D, C, c, E, e are the most important ones. The terms Rh positive, or Rh negative refers to the D antigen only. Those who do have it are Rh positive, and those who don't are Rh negative.

4.6) Lymph nodes

Lymph nodes are organs of the immune system distributed widely throughout the body and linked by lymphatic vessels. They act as filters or traps for foreign particles. They become inflamed or enlarged in various conditions, which may range from a throat infection, to life-threatening situations such as cancer. Lymph enters the lymphatic vessels from the interstitial spaces and then travels to the nodes. Lymph which leaves a node is particularly reach in white blood cells, and will finally drain to the venous system, and return to the hurt.

Lymph Capillaries in the Tissue Spaces

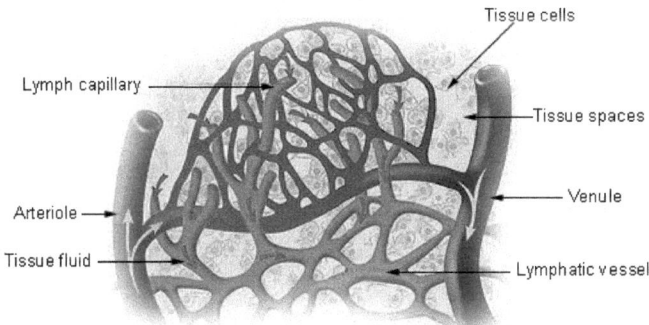

4.7) Heart

The heart is a muscular organ which is located anterior to the vertebral column and posterior to the sternum. The cardiac muscle beats under the influence of the autonomic nervous system and appears cross striated, when a section is observed under the microscope. The human heart is about the size of a fist and has a mass of between 250 and 350 grams. It is enclosed in a double-walled sac called the pericardium. This sac protects the heart, anchors to the surrounding structures, and prevents to some extent, overfilling of the heart with blood. The outer wall of the human heart is composed of three layers. The outer layer is called the epicardium, the middle layer myocardium, and the inner layer endocardium. In a cross section the hurt shows four chambers: two atriae (superior chambers), and two ventricles (inferior chambers). These chambers are divided with valves. Between the right atrium and the right ventricle is the tricuspid valve, and between the right ventricle and the pulmonary artery is the semilunar valve (pulmonary valve). Between the left atrium and the left ventricle is the bicuspid valve (mitral valve), and between the left ventricle and aorta is the semilunar valve (aortic valve).

The flow of the blood through the heart has as follows: deoxygenated blood from the body comes through superior vena cava (head, neck, upper arms), and inferior vena cava (rest of the body), and empties into the right atrium. From here passes to the right ventricle, and then through the pulmonary artery goes to the lungs for oxygenation. Now, oxygenated blood returns through the pulmonary veins to the left atrium. From here passes to the left ventricle and trough it empties into the aorta for systemic distribution. So, in the human body we can distinguish two types of circulation: major (systemic), and minor (pulmonary). Although the heart is full of blood, paradoxically it can't use that blood for its own nourishment, and it needs a special type of circulation. This is called coronary circulation, and through the coronary vessels it provides nourishment and oxygen only to the heart muscle. These vessels have their origin to the aorta and empty into the right atrium (with the rest of the blood).

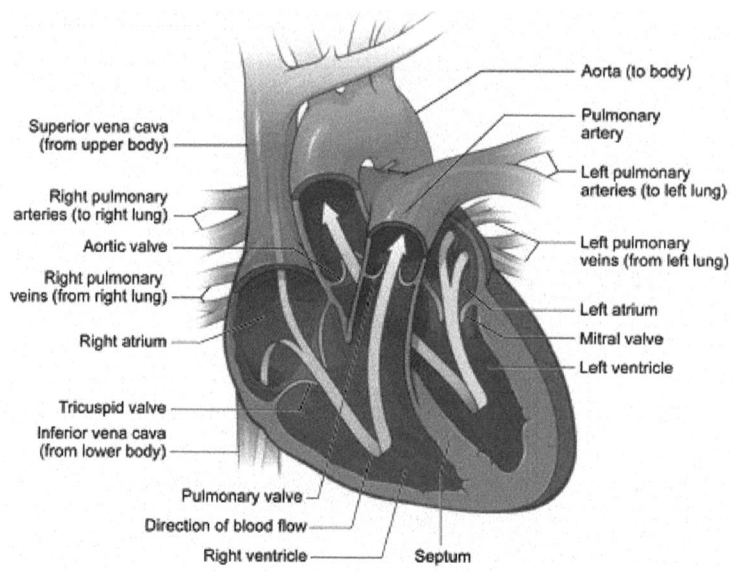

4.8) Lungs

The lungs are essential respiratory organs which transport oxygen from the atmosphere into the bloodstream, and release carbon dioxide from the bloodstream into the atmosphere. They are located in the chest cavity and are indirectly connected with it. From the outside the lungs are covered by a membrane layer, the visceral pleura. This is connected through pleural fluid to the parietal pleura which is

directly connected to the chest wall. So, when the chest wall expands (inspiration), the parietal pleura expand as well. This, due to hydrostatic pressure of the pleural fluid, causes also the visceral pleura to expand, and in this way finally the lungs expand as well. The lungs are also important for the production of the angiotensin converting enzyme. This enzyme converts angiotensin to its active form producing thus the active angiotensin (constriction of the vessels).

We can do physiological measurements so as to estimate the lung's function: 1) Vital capacity, which is the maximum volume of air that a person can exhale after maximum inhalation, 2) Respiratory minute volume, which is the volume of air inhaled, or exhaled in one minute, and at rest is 7-9 liters of air, 3) Respiratory frequency, which is the number of breaths per minute, and at rest is 14-18 breaths/minute.

4.9) Thyroid, parathyroid glands

Thyroid gland is one of the largest endocrine glands in the human body. It is found in the neck region, inferiorly to the thyroid cartilage (Adam's apple), and consists of two lobes (right and left) connected via an isthmus. Its function is controlled by the hypothalamus and hypophysis and produces the hormones: thyroxine (T4), triiodothyronine (T3), and calcitonin. T3 and T4 are synthesized by iodine and tyrosine and participate in the rate of metabolism, growth, and functions of many organ systems in the body. Calcitonin, participates in calcium homeostasis of the body. In response to an increased plasma calcium concentration, secreted calcitonin tries to reduce that level, by several mechanisms, such as deposition of calcium into bones leading thus to their mineralization.

Overactivation of the thyroid gland can lead to hyperthyroidism. This is a metabolic disorder which affects also the sympathetic nervous system. Thus every function of the body tends to speed up; with as a consequence acceleration of the heart rate, tremors of the hands, anxiety, weight loss, muscular weakness, and low cholesterol levels in the blood. In women this condition may affect the menstrual cycle, with less menstrual flow, and menstrual periods occurring less often.

Hypoactivation of the thyroid gland can lead to hypothyroidism. It manifests as cretinism in infants, and myxedema in adults. Clinical manifestations are poor muscular tone, fatigue, cold intolerance, depression, osteoporosis, gain of weight, and bradycardia.

Parathyroid glands are small endocrine glands found behind the thyroid gland. They produce a hormone, parathormone (PTH). Its role is antagonistic to that of the thyroid hormones, and is secreted in response to a low concentration of calcium level in blood plasma. It tries to elevate the calcium level by a variety of mechanisms such as activation of osteoclasts (which will break down parts of the bone so as to release calcium), increased production of vitamin D, increased absorption from the gastrointestinal tract, and increased absorption from the kidneys.

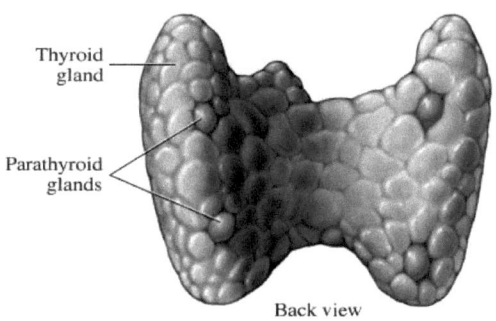

Back view

4.10) Liver

Liver is a vital organ of the human body which is located in the right upper quadrant of the abdominal cavity, resting just below the diaphragm. Its basic structural and functional units are the hepatocytes which are arranged into hepatic lobules. Each hepatic lobule has a central vein and in the periphery carries an arteriole, venule, bile duct, and lymphatic vein. It receives blood from the portal vein (from spleen, gastrointestinal tract and associated organs), and hepatic arteries from the aorta. The liver functions are glycogen storage (reserve of glucose), gluconeogenesis (production of glucose from amino acids and lipids), decomposition of red blood cells, storage of vitamins, iron and copper, conversion of toxic ammonia to urea, synthesis of plasma proteins, detoxification of toxic substances e.g. drugs, and synthesis of angiotensinogen (a hormone which is converted to angiotensin with the aid of angiotensin converting enzyme, produced in lungs). It also helps to the emulsification of dietary lipids, through bile, which is secreted from its gallbladder.

Liver has a remarkable capacity of regeneration and is able to function with only a 25% of its parenchyma. Several disorders of its function such as hepatitis, and cirrhosis may lead inexorable to death, due to incapacity of other organ systems to supplement for its function.

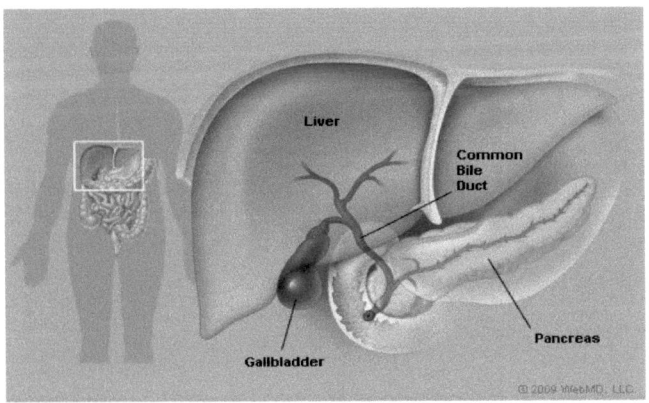

4.11) Pancreas

Pancreas is a compound gland with both an exocrine and endocrine function. The endocrine gland of pancreas consists of the islets of Langerhans. Four cell types exist in these islets: α cells which secrete glucagon, β cells which secrete insulin, δ cells which secrete somatostatin, and PP cells which secrete pancreatic polypeptide.

Glucagon is responsible for raising the blood glucose level by a variety of ways such as: increase gluconeogenesis and β oxidation of fatty acids. This is needed when there is luck of glucose in the blood, or the organism is under stress.

Insulin is mainly secreted after a meal and its main role is to reduce the blood glucose level by leading glucose into the cells where it is stored as glycogen (if there is excess of glucose), or oxidated for production of energy. Luck of insulin may lead to metabolic disorders collectively known as Diabetes mellitus.

Somatostatin inhibits insulin and glucagon secretion. It affects neurotransmission and cell proliferation.

Pancreatic polypeptide regulates the endocrine and exocrine secretion activities of pancreas.

The exocrine gland of pancreas produces digestive enzymes (pancreatic juice) which are secreted into the small intestine. These are trypsin, chymotrypsin, pancreatic lipase, and pancreatic amylase.

Trypsin is a protease enzyme which hydrolyses the proteins.

Chymotrypsin hydrolyses proteins as well.

Pancreatic lipase degrades dietary lipids. This is done by the help of bile which emulsifies the lipids. After emulsification the lipids have a greater area, on which the enzyme can act.

Pancreatic amylase breaks down starch.

4.12) Salivary glands

The oral cavity is associated with three pairs of major salivary glands and a lot of minor salivary glands. Both types are producing saliva which has an extraordinary importance in maintenance of human oral health. Saliva contains an α-amylase which starts the degradation of the dietary starch. It also contains lysozyme and lactoferrin which have bactericidal and bacteriostatic effects, providing thus a barrier for the entrance of microbes to the rest of the body. It has a positive effect in reducing the incidence of dental carries by non permitting the overgrowth of our oral normal flora, and contributes to the mechanical cleansing of the oral cavity. It finally helps in deglutition and speech. The importance of normal salivary flow is highlightened in patients with Sjogren's syndrome (a degenerative disease of the salivary glands).
The major salivary glands are the parotids, submandibular, and sublingual.

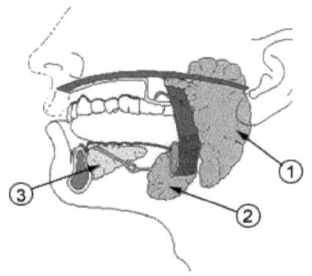

1)   Parotid gland
2)   Submandibular gland
3)   Sublingual gland

4.13) Gastrointestinal tract

The gastrointestinal tract or digestive system is composed of multiple parts and its final role is to provide the body with all the necessary nutrients for its survival and growth. The alimentary canal starts from the mouth where there is some processing of the food through mastication and the action of salivary enzymes. After that the food bolus passes to the pharynx and from here continuous to the esophagus. The esophagus ends to the stomach. The stomach is a muscular, hollow, dilated part of the alimentary canal which can receive a maximum of 1.5-2 liters of food and liquids. It is divided into four parts: the cardia (which receives and temporarily stores the food bolus), the fundus, the body or corpus, and the pylorus with its pyloric sphincter which controls the emptying of the stomach into the small intestine. The epithelium of the stomach wall contains several glands which participate in the digestion process. Every gland has four distinct segments which from the bottom to the top are: 1) enteroendocrine cells which secrete hormone, 2) chief cells which secrete pepsinogen (a precursor of pepsin which is activated in the acidic environment of the stomach and degrades proteins), 3) parietal cells which secrete HCL and intrinsic factor (necessary for the absorption of vitamin B12), 4) mucous neck cells which secrete mucin, protecting thus the stomach wall from its acid contents. The movements of the stomach wall are mixing the food with the gastric juice producing the chyme which is then passed to the small intestine.

The small intestine is 4-5 m long and can be divided into three parts: duodenum, jejunum, and ileum.

The duodenum as the first segment of the small intestine, receives the gastric contents. The duodenal epithelium is releasing secretin and cholecystokinin which causes the release of bile (from liver), and pancreatic enzymes into the duodenum. This causes the neutralization of the acidic chyme and its further digestion.

The jejunum is the mid section of the small intestine. Its inner surface has a mucous membrane which is strongly folded producing thus the intestinal villi. These villi increase the surface area which comes into contact with digested food, increasing thus the absorption of nutrients and water.

The ileum is the final segment of the small intestine. Its main function is the absorbance of vitamin B12 and bile salts.

The large intestine (colon) is 1.5 m long and is divided into: cecum, ascending colon, transverse colon, descending colon, sigmoid colon, rectum and anal canal. Its main function is the absorbance of water and salts and the elimination of the waste products. In the colon there is found the commensal flora which is composed of fermentative and saprogenic bacteria. This flora is beneficial for the host because it digests food residues that the organism cannot on its own, and also repress the growth of potentially harmful microorganisms. They also produce vitamin K which is then absorbed by the organism. Finally, they promote intestinal epithelial cells growth and proliferation. The movement through small and large intestine is achieved by the peristaltic movements of the bowel which are causing the contents to move forward.

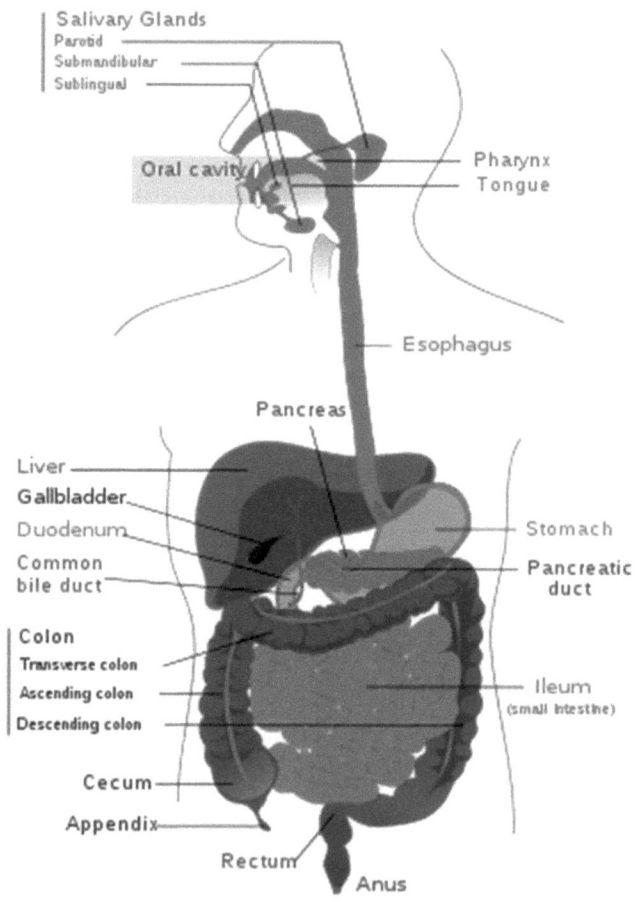

4.14) Kidneys

The kidneys are paired organs found in the abdominal cavity, in the retroperitoneum. The parenchyma of the kidney is divided into a superficial cortex, and a deep medulla. This parenchyma is organized into several renal lobes which are formed from renal cortex and a portion of renal medulla (the renal pyramid). Between the pyramids are projections of the renal cortex, which are called renal columns. The basic structural and functional unit of a kidney is the nephron. Each kidney contains approximately one million nephrons. Their major function is to regulate the concentration of water and soluble substances by filtering the blood, reabsorbing what is needed and excreting the rest as urine. Thus they control blood volume, blood pressure, electrolytes, metabolites and pH of the body. Each nephron is composed from a renal corpuscle (glomerulus and Bowman's capsule), proximal tubule, loop of Henle, and distal tubule. From here a lot of nephrons empty in the same collecting duct. The collecting ducts empty to the renal papillae.

The glomerulus has a filtrate which is identical to the human plasma but without proteins (proteins are very important for the organism so they must be sufficiently holded).

The proximal tubule is concerned with the reabsorption of water and salts, as well as organic solutes (glucose, amino acids).

The loop of Henle is a U shaped tube whose primary function is to reabsorb salts from the filtrate.

The distal tubule actively pumps ions and it is under the influence of the endocrine system. For example, when the organism needs more calcium, the parathyroid hormone causes the distal tubule to actively absorb the calcium ions. At the end of the tubule only 1% water of the initial filtrate remains and the remaining salt content is negligible.

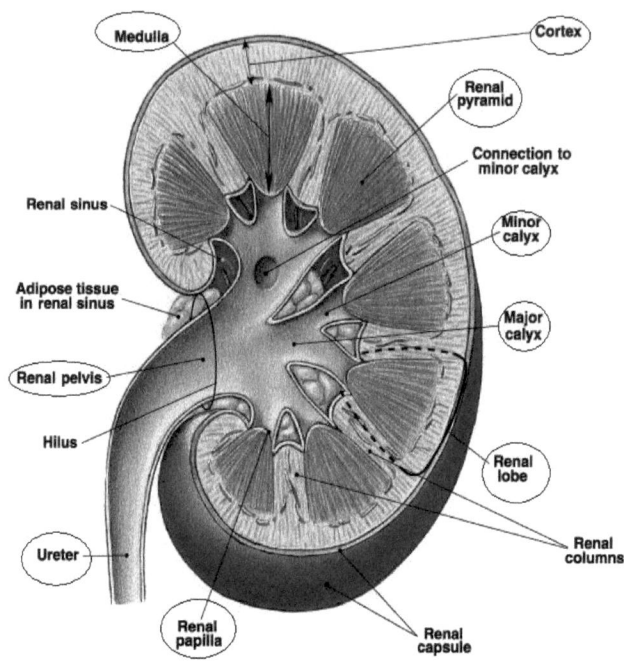

4.15) Suprarenal glands

Suprarenal or adrenal glands are endocrine glands, which sit like a cap over each kidney. They consist of the adrenal cortex and the adrenal medulla. In the adrenal cortex are produced glucocorticoids (mainly cortisol), mineralocorticoids (mainly aldosterone), and adrogens (testosterone). In the adrenal medulla are produced epinephrine (adrenaline) and norepinephrine (noradrenaline).

Cortisol is an antiinflammatory hormone and weakens the immune's system response (that's why it is given after a transplantation so as the immune system will not reject the received organ).

Aldosterone increases sodium and water reabsorption from the kidneys, increasing thus blood volume, and therefore blood pressure.

Testosterone produced in the adrenals is in a very low concentration compared to that produced in testes, and therefore of little significance.

Catecholamines (epinephrine, norepinephrine) are part of the sympathetic nervous system and released in response to stress.

Adrenal Gland

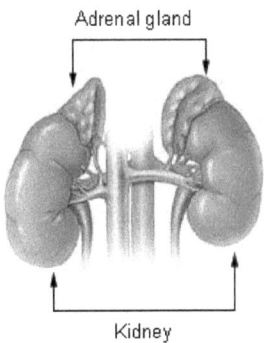

Adrenal gland

Kidney

4.16) Ovaries and menstrual cycle

Ovaries are part of the female reproductive system and act both as gonads and endocrine glands. At birth ovaries contain approximately two million immature follicles from which will reach to puberty only about 500 follicles. Ovaries secrete estrogen and progesterone. Estrogen is responsible for the appearance of secondary sex characteristics of females at puberty, and for the maturation and maintenance of the reproductive organs. Progesterone as the name implies, is a hormone secreted before a potential pregnancy (gestation in Latin means pregnancy). It promotes cyclic changes in the endometrium preparing it thus for a potential pregnancy, and also maintains the endometrium in a healthy state during gestation.

Menstrual cycle can be divided into four phases: proliferative, ovulation, luteal or secretory phase, and menstruation.

During the proliferative phase the secretion of estrogen causes the maturation of a Graafian follicle (it is a follicle inside ovaries which contains fluid and a mature oocyte), and the growth of the uterine mucosa for the implantation of the zygote if the fertilization occur.

During the ovulation the Graafian follicle ruptures and the ovum is released into the oviduct (Fallopian tube). Here it is the place of fertilization with spermatozoon and the production of the zygote. This must be done in a 24 hours period, because after that the ovum disintegrates. In place of the ruptured Graafian follicle is formed the corpus luteum.

During the luteal phase the corpus luteum produces significant amounts of progesterone. If fertilization will not occur the levels of progesterone will fall, and that will trigger menstruation. If fertilization does occur then the developing embryo will produce human chorionic gonadotropin which will preserve corpus luteum. This hormone is produced exclusively from the embryo and thus the pregnancy tests are based on the presence of that hormone.
Menstruation is the shedding of the endometrium which is followed by bleeding of the uterus and the vagina.

4.17) Testes

Testes are part of the male reproductive system and act both as gonads and endocrine glands. Their function begins in puberty and is carried out until old age. They are mainly concerned with the production of spermatozoa and male sex hormones (testosterone). Testosterone promotes the appearance of male secondary sexual characteristics such as an increase in bone and muscle mass, and hirsutism.
The function of testes is controlled by hypophysis through luteinizing hormone (LH), and follicle-stimulating hormone (FSH).

4.18) Hypothalamus, Hypophysis

Hypothalamus is part of the brain (central nervous system) and one of its most important functions is to link the nervous and endocrine system via the hypophysis. It synthesizes releasing hormones which act on the anterior lobe of hypophysis, promoting thus the release of hypophyseal hormones. It also synthesizes antidiuretic hormone (ADH), and oxytocin which travel down to the posterior lobe of hypophysis from where are secreted. Hypothalamus controls body temperature, hunger, thirst, fatigue, and circadian cycles.

Hypophysis (pituitary gland) is divided into three parts: 1) anterior hypophysis (adenohypophysis, or anterior pituitary), 2) posterior hypophysis (neurohypophysis, or posterior pituitary) and 3) intermediate lobe.

Adenohypophysis produces and secretes the following hormones: adrenocorticotropic hormone, ACTH, (controls the function of adrenal cortex), thyroid stimulating hormone, TSH, (controls the function of thyroid gland), prolactin, PRL, (controls the production of milk by the breast), endorphins (endogenous opioids which cause analgesia), growth hormone, GH, (which stimulate the growth), follicle stimulating hormone, FSH, (control the function of testes and ovaries), luteinizing hormone, LH, (control the function of testes and ovaries).

Neurohypophysis stores and releases oxytocin, and antidiuretic hormone, ADH. These hormones are produced in hypothalamus but are secreted from the hypophysis. Oxytocin triggers the contraction of uterus during childbirth so as to facilitate labor, and also triggers the ejection of milk from the mammary glands. Antidiuretic hormone acts on kidney thereby promoting reabsorption of water when the body is dehydrated, and also causes peripheral vasoconstriction thereby increasing blood pressure.

Intermediate lobe is located between the anterior and posterior pituitary. It produces melanocyte-stimulating hormone (MSH). This hormone stimulates the production and release of melanin (melanogenesis) by melanocytes in skin and hair.

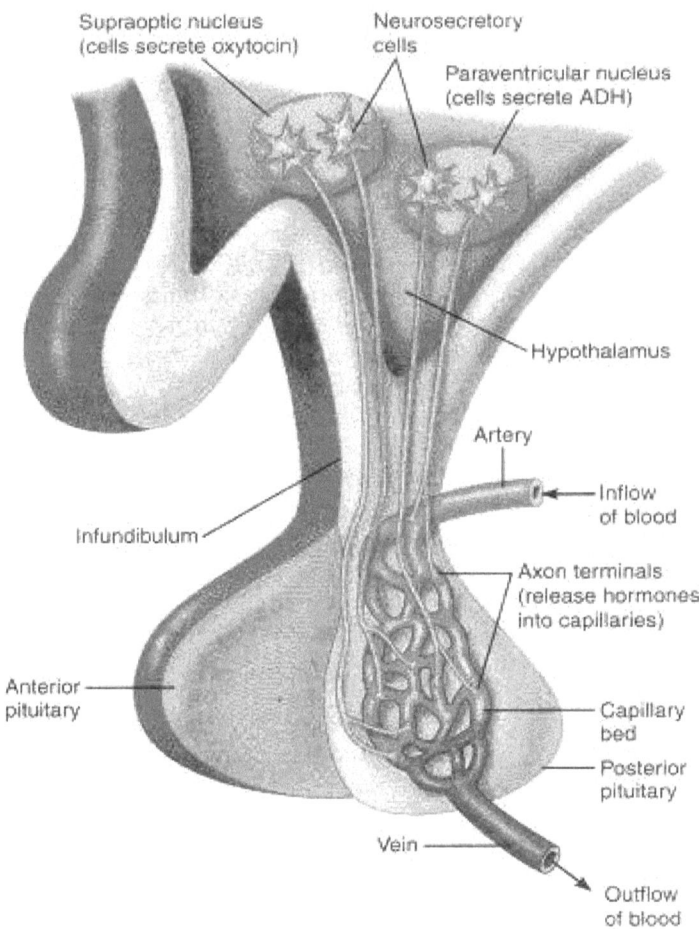

Supraoptic nucleus
(cells secrete oxytocin)

Neurosecretory
cells

Paraventricular nucleus
(cells secrete ADH)

Hypothalamus

Artery

Inflow
of blood

Infundibulum

Axon terminals
(release hormones
into capillaries)

Anterior
pituitary

Capillary
bed

Posterior
pituitary

Vein

Outflow
of blood

4.19) Autonomic nervous system

Autonomic nervous system, as the name implies, is concerned with the autonomic functions of the human body, which are not thus subjected to our will. Its role is to regulate the functions of the human body, in accordance with the external environment, so as to keep its homeostasis. It is part of the peripheral nervous system and is categorized into two groups: parasympathetic nervous system, and sympathetic nervous system. The basic pathway of function of the autonomic nervous system is through a sensory neuron (afferent neuron, goes towards the central nervous system), and a motor neuron (efferent, goes from the central nervous system towards periphery). Thus through the sensory neuron the body senses its environment and passes this information to the central nervous system for processing. After procession the motor neuron carries the response of the central nervous system to the target organ. Sympathetic and parasympathetic divisions typically function in opposition to each other. But this opposition is better understood as complementary rather than antagonistic. For example, when someone is running his heart rate will be increased, under the influence of the sympathetic division. When he will stop the running his heart rate will return back to normal due to the influence of the parasympathetic division.

Parasympathetic nervous system is located in the cervical and sacral regions of the spinal cord. The sensory neurons relies to it information from the environment (external or internal). The motor neurons are divided into preganglionic (before the ganglion) and postganglionic (after the ganglion). The ganglion where preganglionic and postganglionic neurons synapse, is close to the organ of innervation. Parasympathetic nervous system promotes rest and anabolism in the human body. Its functions, in different organ systems are listed as: 1) after optic or olfactory sensation it triggers the secretion of saliva and increases peristalsis. Thus by a simultaneous dilatation of blood vessels which lead to the gastrointestinal tract, it promotes digestion and absorbance of nutrients (anabolism), 2) it causes constriction of the bronchi when the oxygen demands of the body are diminished (at rest), 3) it decrease the heart rate, 4) it causes constriction of the pupil (miosis) and contraction of the ciliary muscles of the lens leading thus to accommodation for a near vision, 5) stimulates sexual arousal.

Sympathetic nervous system is located in the thoracic and lumbar regions of the spinal cord. The sensory neurons relies to it information from the environment (external or internal). The motor neurons are divided into preganglionic and postganglionic. The ganglia are located in the paravertebral ganglionc chain (a chain of ganglia near to the vertebral column). Sympathetic nervous system is concerned with 'fight or flight' reactions. It is activated under the influence of stress and its functions in different organ systems are listed as: 1) diverts the blood flow away from the gastrointestinal tract and skin (through vasoconstriction) and sends it to vital organs, 2) inhibits peristaltic movements of the bowel, 3) constricts all the intestinal sphincters and the urinary sphincter 4) increases blood flow to the skeletal muscles and lungs, 5) dilates bronchioles of lungs allowing thus a greater alveolar exchange between air and blood, 6) increases heart rate and contractility leading thus to an increased cardiac output, 7) causes vasodilation of the coronary vessels of the heart (for better nourishment of the intensively working myocardium), 8) causes dilatation of the pupil and relaxation of the ciliary muscles of the lens, leading thus to accommodation for far vision.

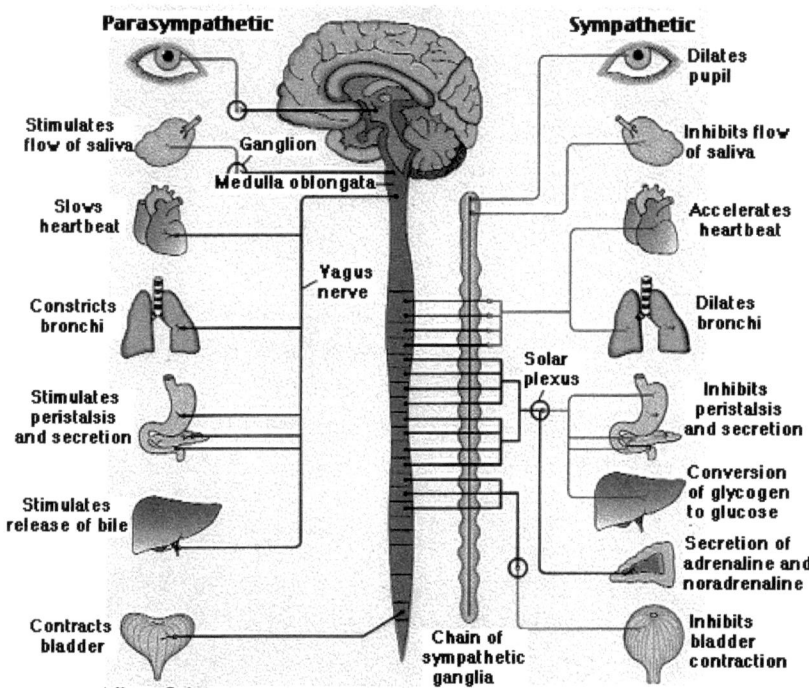

4.20) Vitamins

Vitamins are organic compounds that are required from the human body as nutrients, in small amounts (micronutrients). Except of participating to the nutritional status of an organism they act also as coenzymes (help enzymes in their work), and components of nucleic acids. They can be classified into two groups: fat soluble vitamins (A, D, E, K), and water soluble vitamins (B, C). Fat soluble vitamins they are absorbed with the aid of lipids and they can be stored in the human body. This mast be taken into account because high doses of them can lead to hypervitaminosis (vitamin poisoning). Water soluble vitamins dissolve easily in water and they cannot be stored in the human body (they are excreted through urine). Thus the organism is dependent upon their continuous supply.

Vitamin A (retinol) is regulator of cell and tissue growth and differentiation. It is also found as a pigment of the retina of the eye (rhodopsin). Its deficiency leads to night blindness.

Vitamin B1 (thiamine) functions as coenzyme and is essential for the metabolism of saccharides. Its deficiency leads to Beriberi disease (a nervous system disease)

Vitamin B2 (riboflavin) functions as coenzyme. Its deficiency leads to ariboflavinosis (a condition characterized by anemia, swelling of the mouth and throat mucosa).

Vitamin B3 (niacin) functions as coenzyme. Its deficiency leads to pellagra (a condition characterized by diarrhea, dermatitis and dementia).

Vitamin B4 (adenine) functions as nucleotide base. Its deficiency leads to decreased production of nucleic acids.

Vitamin B5 (pantothenic acid) functions as coenzyme. Its deficiency leads to paresthesia (sensation of pins and needles on the skin of a person).

Vitamin B6 (pyridoxal) functions as coenzyme. Its deficiency leads to anemia and peripheral neuropathy.

Vitamin B7 (biotin) functions as coenzyme. Its deficiency leads to dermatitis and enteritis.

Vitamin B8 (biotin) functions as coenzyme. Its deficiency leads to pins and needles on the skin, and muscular weakness.

Vitamin B9 (folic acid) functions as coenzyme. Its deficiency leads to birth defects such as spina bifida and anencephaly.

Vitamin B10 (factor R). Its deficiency leads to depression and nervousness.

Vitamin B11 (folic acid) functions as coenzyme. Its deficiency leads to child birth problems mentioned before.

Vitamin B12 (cobalamin) functions as coenzyme. Its deficiency leads to anemia.

Vitamin C (ascorbic acid) has antioxidant properties. Its deficiency leads to scurvy. Scurvy presents as defective production of collagen. Collagen appears also in bone tissue and thus its malformation affects bone formation. It also leads to the formation of spots on the skin, spongy gums, and bleeding from the mucous membranes. The spots are most abundant on the thighs and legs. Suppurating wounds (pus forming) and loss of teeth may also be present.

Vitamin D (ergocalciferol) is important for normal absorption of calcium ions from the organism. Its deficiency leads to rickets (softening of bones in children) and osteomalacia (softening of bones in adults).

Vitamin E (tocopherol). Its deficiency leads to anemia.

Vitamin k (phylloquinone) is an 'anti-bleeding' vitamin. Its deficiency leads to bleeding diathesis, which is an unusual susceptibility to bleeding (hemorrhage) due to coagulation dissorders.

References

GENES VIII, Vol. 1, Benjamin Lewin, Pearson Education, Inc.

GENES VIII, Vol. 2, Benjamin Lewin, Pearson Education, Inc.

Principles of Physiology, Matthew N. Levy, Robert M. Berne, Bruce M. Koeppen – 2006

Environmental Physiology of Plants, Alastair H. Fitter, Robert K.M. Hay - 2012

http://media-2.web.britannica.com/eb-media/78/22478-004-521EE704.gif

http://stevebambas.com/images/03_12Exocytosis-L.jpg

http://www.biologie.uni-hamburg.de/b-online/library/biology107/bi107vc/fa99/terry/images/golgi1a.jpg

http://www.biologie.uni-hamburg.de/b-online/library/onlinebio/nucleus_1.gif

http://faculty.ksu.edu.sa/shoeib/Pictures%20Library/06-11_BinaryFission_1.jpg

http://migration.files.wordpress.com/2007/07/eukaryotic-cell.jpg

http://www.life.illinois.edu/ib/335/Vegetative/venation.jpg

http://home.manhattan.edu/~frances.cardillo/plants/angio/cyme2.gif

http://www.biologie.uni-hamburg.de/b-online/library/onlinebio/rootts.gif

http://www.britannica.com/EBchecked/topic-art/602861/1692/Synthesis-of-protein

http://healthbase.files.wordpress.com/2007/06/anatomy-of-spine.jpg

http://www.web-books.com/eLibrary/Medicine/Physiology/Lymphatic/lymph_capillary.jpg

http://www.nhlbi.nih.gov/health/dci/images/heart_interior.gif

http://64.143.176.9/library/healthguide/en-us/images/media/medical/hw/h5550931.jpg

http://www.focalaxis.com/wp-content/gallery/subtle-body/hypothalamus.jpg

http://users.rcn.com/jkimball.ma.ultranet/BiologyPages/A/autonomic.gif

https://www.google.com/search?q=prophase&biw=1350&bih=677&source=lnms&tb
m=isch&sa=X&ved=0ahUKEwjE5LyQxovKAhWC0hoKHYnsA1kQ_AUIBigB#im
grc=4wGz3XA4jDat0M%3A

https://www.google.com/search?q=metaphase&biw=1350&bih=677&source=lnms&t
bm=isch&sa=X&sqi=2&ved=0ahUKEwj37dWNx4vKAhUCtRoKHdzXBCIQ_AUI
BigB#imgrc=ROZiUGXf0JWS_M%3A

https://www.google.com/search?q=anaphase&biw=1350&bih=677&source=lnms&tb
m=isch&sa=X&sqi=2&ved=0ahUKEwjk7uf8x4vKAhXD1BoKHdkLAbgQ_AUIBig
B#imgrc=bdQ27j_PixDu5M%3A

https://www.google.com/search?q=telophase&biw=1350&bih=677&source=lnms&t
bm=isch&sa=X&sqi=2&ved=0ahUKEwjBh_OuyIvKAhWDPBoKHYeeAG4Q_AUI
BigB#imgrc=VP2DVimw_SUCPM%3A

https://www.google.com/search?q=meiosis&biw=1350&bih=677&source=lnms&tb
m=isch&sa=X&sqi=2&ved=0ahUKEwiBnpXwyIvKAhXEVhoKHbSWDYoQ_AUI
BigB#imgrc=6SWtcKT1g9ZidM%3A

https://www.google.com/search?q=eukaryotic+plant+cell&biw=1350&bih=677&sou
rce=lnms&tbm=isch&sa=X&ved=0ahUKEwjfjOX9yYvKAhWInRoKHfn8BasQ_A
UIBigB#imgrc=fVMH802ECjE8FM%3A

https://www.google.com/search?q=carnivorous+plants&biw=1350&bih=677&source
=lnms&tbm=isch&sa=X&ved=0ahUKEwicvavczIvKAhWCVBoKHUcyA0MQ_AU
IBigB#imgrc=P2G-Oly4il9WvM%3A

https://www.google.com/search?q=carnivorous+plants&biw=1350&bih=677&source
=lnms&tbm=isch&sa=X&ved=0ahUKEwicvavczIvKAhWCVBoKHUcyA0MQ_AU
IBigB#tbm=isch&q=leaf+venation&imgrc=TMn8ieNj72q9SM%3A

https://www.google.com/search?q=carnivorous+plants&biw=1350&bih=677&source
=lnms&tbm=isch&sa=X&ved=0ahUKEwicvavczIvKAhWCVBoKHUcyA0MQ_AU
IBigB#tbm=isch&q=scorpioid+cyme&imgrc=wWweR61SdSYGXM%3A

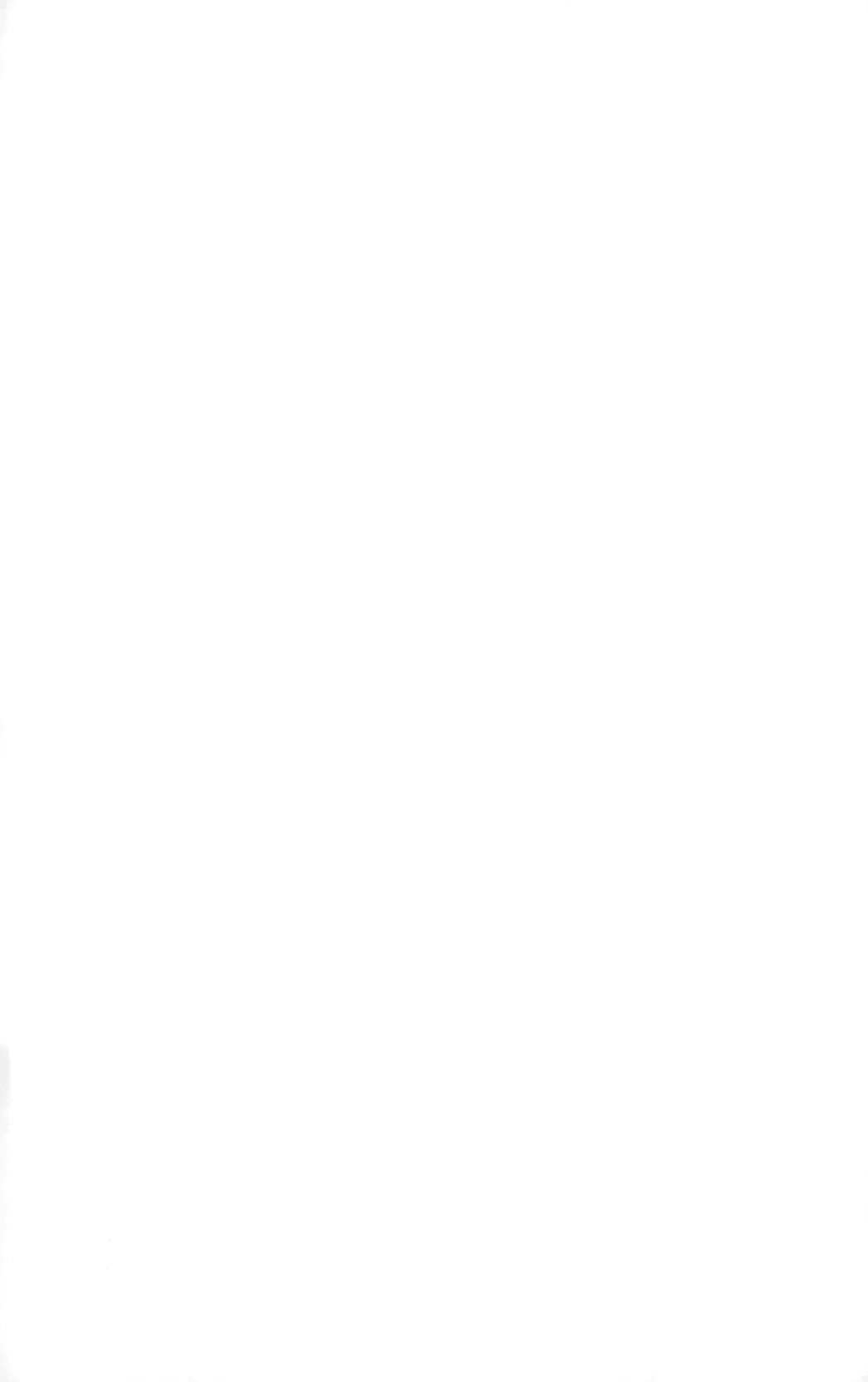

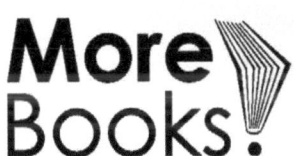
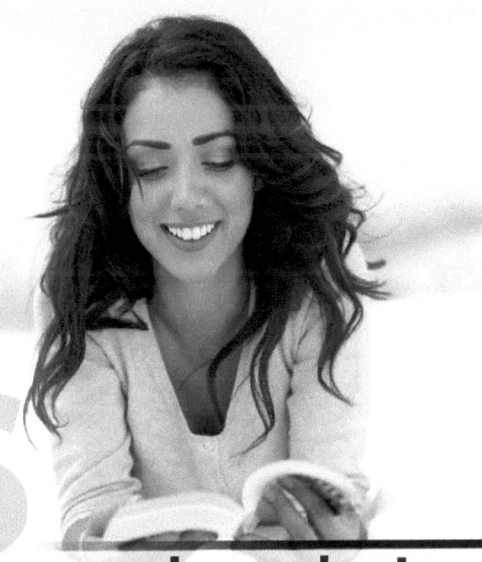
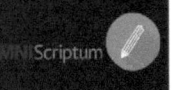

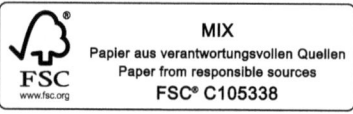
Printed by Books on Demand GmbH, Norderstedt / Germany